Natural Treatments for Arthritis

Overcoming Common Problems Series

Selected titles

A full list of titles is available form Sheldon Press,
36 Causton Street, London SW1P 4ST, and on our website at
www.sheldonpress.co.uk

Asperger Syndrome in Adults
Dr Ruth Searle

The Assertiveness Handbook
Mary Hartley

Assertiveness: Step by step
Dr Windy Dryden and Daniel Constantinou

Backache: What you need to know
Dr David Delvin

Body Language: What you need to know
David Cohen

The Cancer Survivor's Handbook
Dr Terry Priestman

The Chronic Fatigue Healing Diet
Christine Craggs-Hinton

The Chronic Pain Diet Book
Neville Shone

Cider Vinegar
Margaret Hills

The Complete Carer's Guide
Bridget McCall

Confidence Works
Gladeana McMahon

Coping Successfully with Pain
Neville Shone

Coping Successfully with Period Problems
Mary-Claire Mason

Coping Successfully with Prostate Cancer
Dr Tom Smith

Coping Successfully with Psoriasis
Christine Craggs-Hinton

Coping Successfully with Ulcerative Colitis
Peter Cartwright

Coping Successfully with Varicose Veins
Christine Craggs-Hinton

Coping Successfully with Your Hiatus Hernia
Dr Tom Smith

Coping Successfully with Your Irritable Bowel
Rosemary Nicol

Coping When Your Child Has Cerebral Palsy
Jill Eckersley

Coping with Age-related Memory Loss
Dr Tom Smith

Coping with Birth Trauma and Postnatal Depression
Lucy Jolin

Coping with Bowel Cancer
Dr Tom Smith

Coping with Candida
Shirley Trickett

Coping with Chemotherapy
Dr Terry Priestman

Coping with Chemotherapy
Dr Terry Priestman

Coping with Chronic Fatigue
Trudie Chalder

Coping with Coeliac Disease
Karen Brody

Coping with Compulsive Eating
Dr Ruth Searle

Coping with Diabetes in Childhood and Adolescence
Dr Philippa Kaye

Coping with Diverticulitis
Peter Cartwright

Coping with Eating Disorders and Body Image
Christine Craggs-Hinton

Coping with Epilepsy in Children and Young People
Susan Elliot-Wright

Coping with Family Stress
Dr Peter Cheevers

Coping with Gout
Christine Craggs-Hinton

Coping with Hay Fever
Christine Craggs-Hinton

Coping with Headaches and Migraine
Alison Frith

Coping with Hearing Loss
Christine Craggs-Hinton

Coping with Heartburn and Reflux
Dr Tom Smith

Coping with Kidney Disease
Dr Tom Smith

Coping with Life after Stroke
Dr Mareeni Raymond

Overcoming Common Problems Series

Overcoming Common Problems Series

Overcoming Common Problems

Natural Treatments for Arthritis

CHRISTINE CRAGGS-HINTON

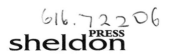

sheldon PRESS

First published in Great Britain in 2011

Sheldon Press
36 Causton Street
London SW1P 4ST
www.sheldonpress.co.uk

The author and publisher have made every effort to ensure that the
external website and email addresses included in this book are correct and
up to date at the time of going to press. The author and publisher are not
responsible for the content, quality or continuing accessibility of the sites.

British Library Cataloguing-in-Publication Data
A catalogue record for this book is available from the British Library

ISBN 978-1-84709-138-3

1 3 5 7 9 10 8 6 4 2

Typeset by Damco Solutions Ltd
Printed in Great Britain by Ashford Colour Press

Produced on paper from sustainable forests

'No one saves us but ourselves. No one can and no one may.
We ourselves must walk the path'

(Buddha)

Contents

Author's note to the reader

This book is intended as a guide to help lower your pain levels and improve your mobility and strength. It also aims to help you cope better emotionally and, all in all, lead a more fulfilling life. It is not a medical textbook and is not intended to replace medical advice. If you think you have arthritis and have not yet consulted your doctor, please do so.

Introduction

Although the main emphasis of this book is natural treatments for osteoarthritis and rheumatoid arthritis, I also discuss juvenile arthritis, fibromyalgia and gout. Note, though, that there are altogether over 200 forms of arthritis, all with several symptoms in common. This book, therefore, should be of use to anyone with any type of arthritis. For the sake of brevity, I refer to all forms of arthritic conditions under the umbrella term of 'arthritis'.

For some, the symptoms of arthritis can range from periodic stiffness and a dull aching, to a near-constant burning pain and disability for others. However, with appropriate management, the person can lead a healthy and independent life. Drug therapy – prescribed by a doctor, pain consultant or rheumatologist – can be invaluable in a flare-up of symptoms, but perhaps the most important treatment of all is self-management. This takes a variety of forms, all of which are discussed in this book.

Morning stiffness is common in arthritis, lasting for at least an hour before it returns to its best state. With a few exceptions, arthritis is inflammatory in nature, causing pain, heat and swelling in one or more joints. If little or nothing is done to halt the progression of the condition, the eventual outcome can be deformity in the affected joints. The condition usually comes on slowly and steadily, but some people experience a sudden acute onset.

The best treatment of arthritis is complex and involves a multi-disciplinary team approach. Physiotherapy is an important component of this as it aims to reduce pain and any inflammation, retain joint mobility, and increase muscle strength. Occupational therapists are also of value as they teach the principles of joint protection, suggest aids to daily living, and advise on adaptations to the home.

Where joint inflammation is accompanied by pain, a doctor will initially prescribe analgesics and anti-inflammatory medication, then move on to drugs called DMARDs that attempt to modify the progression of the condition. I believe there is a place for prescription drugs in the treatment of arthritis for they allow a direct attack on the condition, disrupting its progression and reducing the chances of joint damage and loss of functional ability. Medications are discussed in more detail at the end of Chapter 1.

There is now a firm trend for using natural remedies – usually in combination with prescription medications – and I look at the most common ones in Chapter 2. Certain remedies can be rather expensive, and often there is no scientific evidence to back up the claims of their success. However, some remedies *do* have scientific endorsement and appear to be effective. Chapter 2 can enlighten you as to which ones are most likely to be helpful.

Perhaps the most useful chapters in this book are those offering self-help in both emotional and physical respects – that is, Chapters 3 and 4. Chapter 5 deals with environmental toxins and how they are now known to cause and prolong ill health in those with a genetic predisposition to developing chronic health problems. For instance, did you know that one of the most common chemical sensitivities is to organophosphates, which are now widely used in farming practices throughout the Western world? Organophosphates are highly toxic chemicals used for pest control in crop production and animal husbandry. They are also used in home pesticides such as fly sprays, etc. However, organophosphates were originally developed to attack the central nervous system in order to kill for the purposes of warfare. It is easy to see, then, that they can adversely affect every bodily system. Indeed, they are believed to be implicated in the onset of arthritis and other prolonged conditions.

This leads me nicely into the importance of a low-toxin diet for treating arthritis. Organic foodstuffs, grown without the addition of chemical pesticides and so on, may not always look too appealing, but their taste is superior to non-organic foods. More importantly, rather than being a risk to health, they offer a distinct benefit. Chapter 6, which deals with diet, explains how a healthy balanced diet low in fat and sugar, and high in certain vitamins and minerals, can help to reduce inflammatory flare-ups and therefore assist in normalizing the condition. Non-inflammatory types of arthritis are also likely to respond well to this diet.

Chapter 7 explains how exercise uses up calories that would otherwise be stored as fat, exerting a lot of strain on the joints. Exercise also increases strength and suppleness and is great for good cardiovascular function. I explain how to choose the exercises that are best for you, and each one is accompanied by a diagram and clear instructions. There is also advice on how to build exercise into your daily routine. The last chapter, Chapter 8, discusses posture, explaining how incorrect posture can provoke and prolong pain.

Using self-help techniques (such as mentioned in this book) can make a great difference to your condition – and the more you can help yourself, the better are your chances of improvement. Don't worry if you can only manage to follow a limited amount of my recommendations, for it will be better than nothing – and every little helps. In time, if you try to stay positive and keep my advice in mind, you should be able to help yourself on a much larger scale.

1

What is arthritis?

The word 'arthritis' comes from the Greek *arthro* meaning 'joint' and *itis* meaning 'inflammation'. It describes a group of painful conditions of the joints and/or soft tissues. The word is actually misleading, though, as not all types of arthritis have an inflammatory component. In the same way, although most forms of arthritis are degenerative in nature, this doesn't apply across the board.

As mentioned in the Introduction, there are over 200 types of arthritis, but the most common is osteoarthritis, as discussed in this chapter. The other more prevalent types include rheumatoid arthritis, juvenile arthritis, fibromyalgia and gout.

For many, the pain caused by arthritis is a daily feature, and for some it is almost constant. This is clearly very limiting physically, difficult to cope with on a psychological level, and can severely affect quality of life. Most forms of arthritis swing between times when the pain is aggressively apparent and relatively calmer spells. When the latter is in progress, there may be no pain at all and full mobility restored. For others, however, the calmer times simply mean that the pain reduces to a dull nagging ache. Also, previous severe flare-ups may leave a degree of disability that is always apparent.

Individuals with arthritis would be well advised to learn all they can about it and be involved in their own care. Understanding arthritis is vital in coming to terms with it and helps people to handle the stress and upset it can cause. Moreover, participating in decision-making with healthcare professionals gives back a sense of control and boosts self-esteem. It is also important to be as active as possible, especially when the condition is less aggressive. Indeed, physical exercise is essential if you wish to slow down or halt the progression of arthritis. Exercise options and a number of self-management techniques are described in later chapters.

The history of arthritis

Arthritis has been around for millions of years – even dinosaur bones show evidence of it. Human remains as far back as 4500 BC have shown arthritis to be present; and it was even found in an Italian mummy dating back to 3000 BC, and in Egyptian mummies dating from 2590 BC.

A common condition

An estimated 10–15 million people in the UK are affected by arthritic conditions. This number is expected to rise every year because people in the UK (and elsewhere in the Western world) are living longer, and arthritis – particularly osteoarthritis – is primarily a condition related to ageing. However, people of all ages can develop arthritis, even very young children – although the number of children who have it has not been accurately calculated. Up to the age of 55, men and women are affected equally, but after that, the incidence is higher in women, probably because they are no longer protected by female hormones.

Arthritis is one of the most prevalent long-term health problems in the West, accounting for around 30 per cent of all visits to GPs. Together with heart disease, it is the leading cause of long-term absence from work and the need to claim disability benefits.

Please note that arthritis is not a selective condition. Indeed, it affects all races, ethnic groups and cultures.

A disabling condition

In the UK, a massive 72 per cent of those with arthritis meet the government's 'disability' criteria. This means that several million people with arthritis have difficulties with everyday activities such as bathing, dressing and walking.

Types of arthritis

Although osteoarthritis is by far the main form of arthritis, it can be present in a multitude of other guises, all with pain as the dominant feature. Here are the more common forms:

- RA (rheumatoid arthritis) (see pages 20–3)
- fibromyalgia (see pages 26–30)
- gout (see pages 30–3)

- juvenile arthritis (see pages 23–6)
- lupus
- scleroderma
- bursitis
- psoriatic arthritis
- infectious arthritis
- ankylosing spondylitis (this is inflammation of the spine)
- polymyalgia rheumatica
- Sjögren's syndrome
- tendinitis
- 'nerve trap' conditions – for example, sciatica and carpal tunnel syndrome.

Osteoarthritis

This affects approximately eight million people in the UK. It is more common in women, who tend to be more severely affected, especially in their knees and hands. The condition is characterized by progressive 'wear and tear', causing the gradual deterioration of cartilage – the flexible connective tissue that protects the ends of the joints. Healthy cartilage is very smooth, strong and flexible, but there is a limit to how much wear and tear it can take before it begins to deteriorate, becoming pitted, brittle and thin. As more and more damage to the cartilage occurs, the bones of the joint start to rub together (as discussed on page 7), the result of which is inflammation and pain. This process is also what triggers the development of bony deposits called nodes (or **osteophytes**), as is evident in the knobbly outgrowths on some people's knuckles.

Over time, the bone beneath what is left of the cartilage thickens and becomes broader. This results in the bone capsule being larger in breadth than before, meaning it can hold more synovial fluid – the viscous lubricating substance held in a thick flexible membrane or sac, its function being to lubricate the joint. Any excess of synovial fluid in the joint will then make it swell, causing feelings of stiffness and pain.

The main areas affected by osteoarthritis are the weight-bearing joints, as indicated by arrows in the cartoon on the next page.

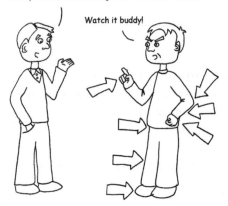

People don't usually get osteoarthritis in all these places at once. One person may have it in their hips and knees, whereas another may have it in their knuckles and toes.

Osteoarthritis is more likely to appear with advancing age, but it usually starts between the ages of 40 and 60. By the age of 70 it is thought that almost everyone has it – even if it only manifests itself as morning stiffness. In some cases, it develops gradually, over many years, and the changes can be so subtle they are hardly noticeable. For others, the condition has a fairly rapid onset and the individual is very aware of increasing pain and restricted movement.

As the course of the condition is impossible to predict, its medical treatment requires a great deal of experience. If, despite medication, permanent joint deformity occurs with accompanying severe pain and reduced mobility, surgery may be the best option. Each year around 60,000 hip replacements and a similar number of knee replacements are carried out in the UK as a result of osteoarthritis. Of course, osteoarthritis can occur in areas of the body that, despite future advances in medical procedures, may always be impossible to 'replace' – such as the spine. Quite often it is feasible, though, to control symptoms by natural means, as discussed in this book. The earlier in arthritis you start helping yourself, the more likely you are to make positive changes. However, it is never too late to help yourself.

As has been previously mentioned, osteoarthritis is the main manifestation of arthritis, with a far higher prevalence than any of the other types. Therefore, osteoarthritis is simply referred to as 'arthritis' much of the time. The other forms of arthritis are generally known by their full names. As this chapter discusses other types of arthritis, I have chosen to give osteoarthritis its full name throughout for the sake of clarity.

Symptoms

As stated, osteoarthritis is a condition that develops over time. It is often so mild at the outset it is easy to miss and may not be noticed until it progresses to distinct aching and stiffness in one or more joints – commonly in the finger joints, knees or hips. This can be confused with the symptoms of injury to the joint, and most people begin by 'treating' themselves, using heat pads and ice packs, rubbing on creams, and taking over-the-counter painkillers. Should such symptoms last for more than two weeks, however, you would be best advised to consult your doctor. A joint injury would almost certainly have improved in that time.

When the condition really starts to take hold, the symptoms develop into what has been described as 'a deep aching pain', and is more evident after engaging in hard work or weight-bearing exercise. Using the affected joint at the end of the day will also make the pain worse, but this is usually relieved by rest. The onset in certain people is so rapid that the pain even interrupts their sleep. Morning stiffness is also common, but this usually eases as the joints loosen with rest, or with gentle use. As the day goes on, pain levels are likely to increase when the affected joints become tired. Limited movement of these joints is also a common problem – even early on in the development of osteoarthritis.

Unless the progression of the condition is interrupted – usually by a combination of medical intervention and self-help measures – symptoms are likely to fluctuate and you are liable to experience flare-ups followed by remissions. The number of flare-ups you have may depend on your weight and posture, as well as how active you are and how much stress is exerted on the affected joints. Gentle activity is nearly always beneficial, but vigorous exercise or repeated weight-bearing activity is usually too much for the joint and likely to provoke a flare-up.

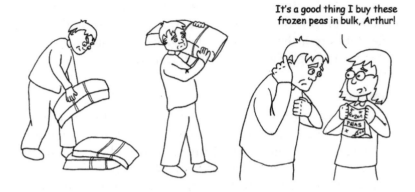

In some people, deforming nodes (osteophytes) appear at the margins of affected joints in the hands (knuckles), and they are often red, hot, swollen and very tender. As a result, there is numbness and loss of dexterity – a significant problem as we use our hands in almost everything we do.

Osteoarthritis in other areas of the body can make it difficult or impossible to walk, bend down, stretch and so on. Some people even need a carer to help them.

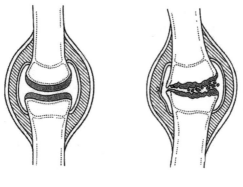

Normal joint   *Advanced arthritis*

Figure 1 A normal joint versus a joint with advanced arthritis

With the passage of time, there may be a grating or catching sensation in the joint during movement – the knees and hips are commonly affected in this way if osteoarthritis continues unhindered. This occurs because a part of the damaged cartilage has broken away from the bone, leaving the ends of the bone exposed. Consequently, the bone ends scrape and abrade against one another, straining and weakening the ligaments in the area, causing a lot of pain and even changing the appearance of the joint. When the joints reach the knobbly stage, however, there is the bonus that they are usually less painful or even pain-free.

Unfortunately, osteoarthritis is a degenerative condition, meaning that it will gradually worsen unless either of the following occurs:

• You take steps to interrupt the progression of the condition.
or:
• The osteoarthritis eventually burns itself out, leaving you either pain-free or with far less pain. However, any deformity to your joints will remain.

As early diagnosis can help to prevent unnecessary damage, it is important that you see your doctor and do not ignore symptoms. Also, the sooner you start to use self-help techniques in combination with drug therapy, the easier it is to slow down or stop the progression of the condition. Figure 1 on the previous page shows a normal joint alongside advanced arthritis in the same joint.

The inflammation of osteoarthritis

As mentioned, most types of arthritis involve a degree of inflammation. Where osteoarthritis is concerned, the inflammation occurs in the cartilage and other soft tissues in the locality of the affected joint. Believing it is being invaded by a foreign substance, the body's immune system triggers the production of masses of protective antibodies called **immunoglobulin E** ('IgE' for short) to mount an attack on the 'invaders'. We all have a number of IgE defenders whose aim it is to fight off these 'invaders', but people who are allergic to certain substances produce too many for their own good when this response is provoked. The result of this sudden overabundance is termed a **systemic inflammatory response**, which means that one of the body's systems – in this case the joints in osteoarthritis – becomes swollen, reddened, hot and often painful.

The pain of osteoarthritis

When nerves in an area affected by inflammation release chemical signals into the brain, they are recognized as pain. Pain is the body's alarm system that tells you that something is

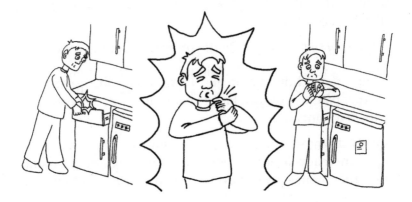

wrong and that you need to act. For instance, if you accidentally trapped your finger in a drawer, pain signals would travel up to your brain and you would respond by quickly opening the drawer and releasing your finger. Ongoing pain would then send you heading to your freezer to look for ice to put on the finger.

The most difficult part of having osteoarthritis (or another form of arthritis) is dealing with the persistent pain. However, you can manage the pain better by seeing it as a signal to take positive action. Of course, it's not always possible to get rid of pain, but there are plenty of things you can do to keep it at bay. These things are discussed at length in the following chapters.

Depression and osteoarthritis

Osteoarthritis (and other forms of the condition) can lead to depression, as demonstrated by Martin and his colleagues in research presented in an abstract to the American College of Rheumatology Annual Scientific Meeting in 2008.[1] During the course of this research, some 2,000 members of the public were questioned about any illnesses they had and asked to assess their pain intensity and physical limitations. Those with arthritis had greater pain and impaired mobility, poorer mental health, less satisfaction with life and more symptoms of depression than most of the others. The conclusion was that persistent pain and mobility problems can cause depression and that pain-management strategies are important in maintaining good mental health.

Risk factors in osteoarthritis

Until recently, osteoarthritis was thought to be an inevitable part of ageing. Indeed, for many years it was described simply as a 'wear and tear' problem. Opinions are changing, however, and doctors now realize that several factors, often in combination, can result in osteoarthritis.

Previous injury

Doctors have known for a long time that major injury can lead to osteoarthritis. The reason for this is that damage to a joint creates irregularities on its previously smooth surface. For example, a fracture of the tibia (one of the two long bones in the lower leg) is likely to mean that a broken area of bone pierces the cartilage protecting the knee joint. This, in turn, triggers further cartilage destruction. The end of the bone is left inadequately protected by cartilage, allowing the bones of the joint to scrape together. The result is the inflammation and pain of osteoarthritis.

In the same way, surgery on a joint can, in later life, lead to osteoarthritis at this site.

Genetics

Evidence indicates that genetic factors play a major role in osteoarthritis – in other words, the condition often runs in the family. Doctors have known for a long time that nodal osteoarthritis (where knobbly growths form on the hands) is genetically linked in some families. In a recent study of identical twins with osteoarthritis, it was found that up to 65 per cent of cases were genetic in nature.

There are rare forms of osteoarthritis that occur in families and start at a young age – and they have been linked to a gene that acts on collagen (the main structural protein found in the connective tissues of joints). Whether the same genetic defect is present in older people with the common form of osteoarthritis is not yet known. Further research is required in this area.

Age

Although advancing age was mentioned earlier as a risk factor, I should add that cartilage becomes more brittle and less capable of repairing itself as the years go by. Therefore, osteoarthritis is more likely to arise the older you become. When osteoarthritis develops in younger people, the reason is usually inherited faulty genes or previous injury.

Being overweight/obese

Damage to a joint is partly dependent upon how much weight it has to support – with the hips, spine and knees of heavier people being particularly at risk. Unless weight is lost and the body mass index (BMI) (see page 100 for a BMI chart) falls to within normal levels, an overweight/obese person stands more chance of getting osteoarthritis, and of the condition worsening once it has developed. It is therefore important to lose excess weight and then keep your weight as close as you can to that recommended for your height.

Eating a balanced diet helps to nourish the muscles, cartilage and bone, reducing the risk of osteoarthritis or slowing down the progression of osteoarthritis once it has started. Note that for every one pound of weight you lose, the load exerted on the knee joints during activity is reduced by four pounds. In some people, the risk of developing osteoarthritis in the knee is cut by half when they lose as few as 11 pounds. If an overweight individual with osteoarthritis loses only 15 pounds, their knee pain should effectively be cut by half.

(See Chapter 6 for more information on nutrition to help with arthritis, and the Useful addresses section for details of a weight loss company.)

Physically demanding jobs

People who work in heavy construction or do arduous repetitive work where a particular joint (or set of joints) is involved stand a greater chance of developing osteoarthritis than people who have 'lighter' jobs.

Illness and infection

Osteoarthritis can also occur as a result of the following:

- a septic infection in a joint
- repeated episodes of gout
- rheumatoid arthritis in one or more of the joints.

In addition, there are several other medical conditions that can inflame the joints and lead to osteoarthritis.

Participating in sport

Normal activities such as walking and swimming, together with participating in many sports, are generally very good for the joints. It is only when the activity or sport is very 'aggressive' to the body (for example, rugby), causing undue physical stress or a risk of injury to a joint, that osteoarthritis can result over time. The risk is greater if exercise is resumed too soon after injury, before the joint has had time to fully repair itself. If you experience an injury, you should ask your doctor or physiotherapist when it is safe to recommence a sport or activity.

Please note that the benefits of being generally active are thought to outweigh the risk of injury. However, if you partake in an aggressive sport such as rugby and frequently get injured, it would obviously be safer for you in the long term to take up a less vigorous activity.

Chemical sensitivities

Some allergy specialists believe there is a link between osteoarthritis and environmental toxins, which can be highly allergenic. It was actually Dr Theron Randolph of Chicago who first noticed great improvements in many people who made an effort to remove pollutants from their environment and certain foods from their diet (foods to which they had already displayed an intolerance reaction). See Chapter 5 for information on decreasing the amount of indoor and outdoor air contaminants you are exposed to, and Chapter 6 for removing chemicals from your diet.

Weather conditions

Although certain weather conditions seem to temporarily affect the symptoms of osteoarthritis, they can not cause the condition or add to its progression. People with osteoarthritis (and other types of arthritis) often say that their joints ache more than normal when the atmospheric pressure is falling and the air is more humid – that is, just before a storm or heavy rainfall. There is little scientific evidence to support these claims – but, having said this, people are often very accurate in their predictions with regard to this.

Interestingly, there are no fewer cases of osteoarthritis in warmer regions of the world than in colder ones. People who live in a warmer climate are more likely to take regular exercise, though, which can halt the progress of arthritis.

Getting a diagnosis

As experts believe that joint destruction begins within the first two years of developing arthritis, getting an early diagnosis can help to prevent unnecessary damage. It's important, therefore, that you see your doctor as soon as you think there is a problem. From your answers to his or her questions and a physical examination, the doctor will be able to decide whether or not your symptoms are a result of osteoarthritis, a sports injury or another condition entirely.

The following are questions the doctor is likely to ask you:

- What are your symptoms?
- When and how did they start?
- How have they changed over time?
- How do they interfere with your work and daily life?
- Do you have any other health problems?
- Do you take any medications?

If you tend to get a little flustered in the doctor's surgery, it might be best to write down the answers to these questions and have them to hand on a piece of paper when you go in. Remember to give your doctor a clear description of your pain, stiffness, swelling and any mobility problems.

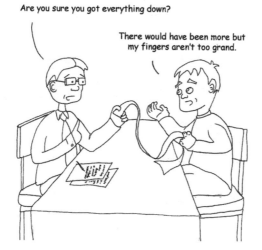

Your doctor will examine the areas of your body affected, feeling for bony swellings, restricted movement, joint tenderness, creaking joints, thinning muscle, excess fluid and instability in the joints.

X-rays

Although there is as yet no blood test to diagnose osteoarthritis, your doctor may order such tests to rule out other conditions. Perhaps the most useful test for diagnosing osteoarthritis and checking the amount of joint damage is the humble X-ray, which uses electromagnetic waves of high energy and very short wavelength. These waves are able to pass through the many constituents of the body and create a photographic image of the skeletal structure. An X-ray will also show the degree of cartilage loss, bone damage and nodule growth. They are not able to reveal the future course of the condition, of course – in other words, how much of a problem it is likely to be in the future. Very early osteoarthritis damage will not show up on X-rays either.

MRI scanners

Although researchers believe that X-rays give sufficient information for the diagnosis of osteoarthritis, some doctors send their patients to a hospital for magnetic resonance imaging (MRI) scans. Since X-rays are far cheaper than an MRI scan,

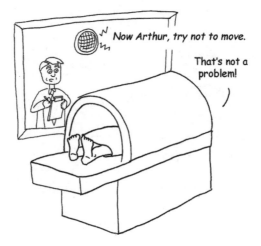

deciding which to use has become a bone of contention in the medical world.

MRI machines use radio waves and a strong magnetic field to look inside the human body. The individual lies on a retractable platform which takes him or her inside a large scanning machine. Several magnetic coils emitting a radio frequency pulse are aimed at the painful area, disturbing hydrogen atoms within the body. It is as the atoms relax that the computer attached to the scanner receives messages that make up a picture.

X-rays and MRI scans are both painless procedures.

Joint aspiration 1

If there is swelling, pain and stiffness in one or more of the joints, a doctor may decide to draw off some of the fluid – a process called **joint aspiration** (see page 17). The fluid is then sent to a laboratory for examination.

This procedure not only makes a painful area more comfortable, it also aids diagnosis.

You and your doctor

To ensure you are offered the most effective treatment possible, it is important that you develop a good relationship with your doctor. This can only happen if you are able to:

- tell your doctor exactly how you are feeling;
- explain how osteoarthritis is affecting your life;
- ask any questions that pop into your head, no matter how silly they may seem to you – it's better to feel silly than to be in doubt about something.

Medical consultations are invariably more advantageous if you don't allow yourself to feel rushed. You could perhaps book a double appointment (that is, one that is twice as long as the usual ones) so you have more time to relax. As already mentioned, writing things down can help you to give your doctor the whole picture and is a safety measure in case your mind goes blank. You may even wish to take someone with you to the appointment – someone who knows how the condition impinges on your life and can prompt you if you forget to mention something important.

The aim of medical treatment

The treatment offered to a person with osteoarthritis will depend largely upon the severity of their symptoms. It focuses on decreasing pain levels, easing stiffness, and improving joint mobility.

Hospital referrals

At some stage, your doctor will probably refer you to a rheumatologist for specialist advice regarding the medical management of your condition. You may also be referred to a pain specialist or offered a place, along with others who have pain, on a pain-management programme where cognitive behavioural therapy (CBT) is high on the agenda; this type of therapy will help you to acquire techniques for coping with pain. It is also common for a pain specialist to see you in order to instruct you on how best to use your medications.

Surgery

When the pain of osteoarthritis is severe and/or there is a risk of function loss, a surgical procedure known as **arthroplasty** can be your best option. This approach focuses on reconstructing or replacing an affected joint, and is usually successful in restoring mobility. Indeed, most of us know someone who has undergone hip or knee replacement surgery and is now pain-free (or virtually pain-free) and can walk normally once more. Another option is **arthrodesis** – this is a less common procedure where two damaged joints are fused together. A third option is **osteotomy** where the affected joint is surgically realigned. This procedure is usually offered in an area of the body where it is not feasible to replace or fuse joints.

If you are referred to an orthopaedic surgeon, the decision as to whether you wish to go down this route will be yours. It is important, though, before you make any decision, that you feel you have as much information as possible about the pros and cons of any surgical procedure. If you are unsure about anything, don't forget to ask – even if it means making an extra appointment with the surgeon just for that reason.

Joint aspiration 2

When a lot of fluid collects around an inflamed joint, causing pain, swelling and restricted movement, a doctor may **aspirate** the joint to make you more comfortable. Using a syringe, a hollow needle is carefully inserted beneath your skin and into the swollen area. The fluid is then removed by means of suction. Some doctors send drained fluid from a joint for laboratory analysis to assist them in making a diagnosis.

Drug therapy

Although the main focus of this book is treatment by natural means, it would be foolish of me to exclude information about medication in general. Painkillers, anti-inflammatory drugs and so on can help you reach a stage where you are largely able to manage the condition via self-help techniques. They can also stop your condition from progressing, allowing you to lead a more active, pain-reduced life. For the best results possible, many people choose to use a combination of prescription medications and self-management techniques.

Painkillers

Painkillers (also called analgesics) will not improve your osteo-arthritis or affect it in any way, but they can be invaluable for reducing pain to more bearable levels and relieving stiffness. The safest painkiller is **paracetamol**, the lower strengths of which are available over the counter from your local pharmacy or supermarket. Low- and medium-strength paracetamol seldom cause side effects – indeed, the only real risk is liver damage from taking large doses, usually over a prolonged period. Stronger doses of paracetamol, or a combination of paracetamol and a **codeine** compound (which is also a stronger medication), are available only on prescription and carry a greater risk of side effects such as constipation and/or dizziness.

Non-steroidal anti-inflammatory drugs

If some inflammation is present in your joints, you may be pre-scribed a course of non-steroidal anti-inflammatory drugs

(NSAIDs), such as **ibuprofen**, **naproxen**, **piroxicam** or **diclofenac**. This type of drug is non-narcotic, meaning it doesn't affect mood or have tranquillizing properties. NSAIDs can usually reduce inflammation and therefore pain levels. However, there is more likelihood of side effects with this type of drug – for example, diarrhoea and digestive tract problems. NSAIDs are also capable of interacting with other medications, such as drugs for treating high blood pressure and heart disease.

NSAID creams and gels are available over the counter and on prescription, depending upon their strength. Topical NSAID creams include **proflex**, **ibuprofen** and **voltaren**, and should be rubbed into the skin at the site of pain and inflammation two or three times daily, according to instructions on the package or accompanying leaflet. Osteoarthritis in the hands and knees responds particularly well to NSAID creams and gels.

Cox-2 inhibitors

This newer type of NSAID directly lowers levels of an enzyme called Cox-2, a natural chemical in the body that promotes inflammation and pain. Cox-2 inhibitors are also less likely than the normal NSAIDs to cause digestive problems that can lead to the formation of a peptic ulcer. However, researchers suspect that Cox-2 inhibitors carry an increased risk for high blood pressure, heart attack, thrombosis and stroke, particularly when used in high doses for a prolonged period. It was because of these concerns that a Cox-2 inhibitor called Vioxx was voluntarily removed from the market in 2004.

Celecoxib, **etoricoxib**, **parecoxib** and **rofecoxib** are types of Cox-2 inhibitors.

Disease-modifying anti-rheumatic drugs (DMARDs)

DMARDs is a group of immune-suppressant drugs that can effectively slow down the progression of arthritis. Although they seldom result in a complete remission, they do seem to reduce inflammation. Their main function, however, is to slow the progression of the condition by modifying the immune system. A range of studies have shown DMARDs to be very effective, with an exceptionally low risk of serious side effects. Indeed, they are now regarded as a good long-term treatment for controlling symptoms. Types of DMARD include **methotrexate, sulfasalazine** and **hydroxycholoroquine.**

Corticosteroids

When joints are unresponsive to other forms of treatment, a doctor or surgeon may suggest injecting the area with cortico-steroids to give pain relief that can last for up to six months. Steroids are similar to the natural hormones in our bodies that help to reduce inflammation – of course, if inflammation is not a particular problem for you, corticosteroids are not likely to be beneficial. The common side effects linked to cortico-steroids are mood swings, nervousness, insomnia, weight gain, high blood pressure and fluid retention. Less common side effects include muscle weakness, stomach ulcers, glaucoma and acne. Long-term use of this type of drug can have serious side effects, including osteoporosis, easy bruising and thinning of the skin. Corticosteroid injections are not given more than four times a year into a specific joint area.

Examples of corticosteroids are **celestone, depo-Medrol, kenalog** and **aristospan.**

Research developments

There is currently a five-year trial underway – launched at the end of 2010 and funded by Arthritis Research UK – in which stem cells extracted from 70 people with knee osteoarthritis are being mixed with the cells in cartilage, called **chondrocytes.** Stem cells are immature undeveloped cells in bone marrow that can be changed into different kinds of tissue and then grown in a laboratory. Keyhole surgery is used to extract the cells from people, and after appropriate growth they are implanted with chondrocytes into the damaged area of the knee in the hope that repair will be triggered and eventually new cartilage will grow.

Professor Sally Roberts and Professor James Richardson who are running the trial at Keele University are optimistic that the procedure will be successful, reducing the need for surgery and pain-relieving drugs. In 2010, before the start of the trial, they were quoted in the *Daily Telegraph* newspaper as saying, 'They [the combination of stem cells and chondrocytes] certainly have huge potential – we just need to learn how to harness it properly.' Jane Tadman, spokesperson for Arthritis Research UK, was quoted (in the same newspaper) as responding with, 'We think this has great potential, but the trial is experimental and we really need to find if it works before we get too excited.'

There is certainly a great deal of scientific research underway into the different forms of arthritis and it is to be hoped that better drugs and treatments will shortly be available.

Rheumatoid arthritis

Rheumatoid arthritis (RA, for short) is the second most common type of arthritis. However, it is recognized as the most disabling form. The condition affects between one and three per cent of the population in the Western world and can arise at any age – even in childhood. RA is increasingly common with advancing age, but normally begins after the age of 40. Women are two to three times more likely than men to have it, which indicates that oestrogen (the main female hormone) is implicated in its onset and progression.

Researchers are currently looking at the role of oestrogen in RA.

An inflammatory condition

RA is an inflammatory condition that mainly affects the joints and tendons. It causes pain, stiffness, swelling (inflammation) and a sensation of heat in the area. The individual may also feel generally unwell, experiencing feverishness, nausea and tiredness. Inflammation is normally the body's way of healing an injured area, but in RA the immune system mistakenly attacks the body's own tissues instead of defending and repairing them. It is therefore an 'auto-immune' condition.

The inflammation of RA affects:

- the thin membrane (the synovial membrane) that lines the joint capsule – this is the part most commonly affected by RA;

- the protective sheaths (tubes) that surround tendons;
- the fluid-filled sacs (called bursae) that allow the muscles and tendons to move smoothly over one another.

When the synovial membrane is attacked, it becomes sore and inflamed, which triggers the release of a certain group of chemicals. Over time, these chemicals cause the synovial membrane to thicken, damaging bones, cartilage, tendons and ligaments if no action is taken to halt the process. Joint deformity sometimes results, and in a few cases the joint is completely destroyed.

Researchers are currently investigating why it is that a person's immune system can start to attack tissues that it is supposed to protect. Many experts believe that an infection, virus, injury or exposure to environmental toxins can trigger the condition in someone who is predisposed to developing it – and as it tends to run in families, the predisposition is thought to be genetic. Consequently, the theory is that if a triggering event fails to occur, the condition will remain dormant for a lifetime, and the person will never know they were genetically programmed to develop RA. Researchers have, as yet, to single out any genes that may be responsible for causing the predisposition. In the meantime, there is a great deal of scientific interest in families with RA.

RA usually affects more than one joint and can cause problems in any joint in the body. If one hand or knee is attacked by RA, the other is likely to be, too. However, RA affects everyone differently, which makes it difficult to diagnose. There are usually times when the condition is active, provoking a lot of joint pain and mobility problems (referred to as a 'flare-up' or 'relapse') as opposed to times when it improves and there is only mild discomfort (referred to as a 'remission'). The pain and stiffness are usually more apparent in the morning, when the person first gets up, and this usually eases as the day goes on and as the joints are flexed and used.

The symptoms of RA tend to develop gradually with the first indicators being pain and tenderness in the small joints of the fingers or toes. It will often spread to other joints such as the shoulders, elbows, hips and jaw, affecting several areas at once during a flare-up. One in four people with RA develop painless lumps under their skin (called rheumatoid nodules). These nodules usually appear on the skin around the elbows and forearms. Unlike osteoarthritis, RA can cause inflammation in other parts of the body, such as the tear glands, salivary glands, blood vessels and the lining of the heart and lungs.

Some people have RA for only a short period of time before it disappears without causing damage – that is, a few months or a couple of years. Others swing between flare-ups and remissions for many years. A relatively small number of people have a severe form of the condition that can last a lifetime in some cases. With the latter, serious joint damage is likely to occur.

Getting a diagnosis

As many conditions can cause joint inflammation and stiffness, your doctor will need to check the mobility of your joints and look for any swelling. To help him or her reach the correct diagnosis, it is vital that you mention *all* your symptoms – not just the ones that you think are important. As eight out of ten people with RA have a specific antibody in their blood called the 'rheumatoid factor', you are likely to have blood tests. Note, though, that in the early stages of RA not everyone has this antibody. To confuse the matter further, it is actually found in 1 in 20 people who *don't* have the condition.

Treatment

Unfortunately, there is no cure for RA. There are drugs, however, that can relieve the symptoms and even slow its progression. These include painkillers, NSAIDs, Cox-2 inhibitors, cortico-steroids and DMARDs, as discussed earlier in this chapter (see page 18). The latter all work by blocking the chemicals that attack the joints and tendons. As a result, symptoms are eased and the progress of RA slowed down. Note that it can take four to six months before you see positive results.

Surgery

As with osteoarthritis, the procedure known as arthroplasty can be a good option, particularly when the pain has become severe and/or there are mobility problems. With this procedure, an affected joint is reconstructed or replaced and mobility is usually restored. As mentioned earlier, arthrodesis is another surgical procedure that fuses joints together. Unfortunately, not all the joints in the body can be replaced. When this is the case, another type of surgery called osteotomy may be offered to help realign the joint.

Surgery on the joints in the hands is a third option for people with RA. In this procedure, damaged tendons (the strong fibrous material connecting muscle to bone) are repaired to improve hand function.

Please ensure that any questions you may have are answered to your satisfaction before you agree to go ahead with any type of surgery.

Research developments

For many years, researchers have attempted to find the reason for the abnormal immune response in RA, but to no avail so far. As mentioned, scientific theories point to a genetic predisposition and a triggering event.

We can only hope that before too long further research will lead to better treatments and an improved prognosis.

Juvenile rheumatoid arthritis

Juvenile rheumatoid arthritis (JRA) – often simply known as juvenile arthritis – is the term for a group of arthritic conditions affecting children up to the age of 16. They all cause joint stiffness and inflammation and can result in pain, swelling and mobility problems lasting more than six weeks. One or two children per thousand are affected, with 80 per cent of cases resolving after the age of 15, with the child regaining normal function. The prognosis is worse in children who develop JRA before the age of five.

Unfortunately, JRA can result in bone development problems, with the affected joints growing faster or slower than the healthy joints. This can cause obvious deformity, with one arm or one leg ending up shorter than the other. In addition, the joints may grow unevenly, making the limb (or limbs) affected noticeably crooked.

As with adult RA, a child with JRA will experience flare-ups and remissions. Some children have only one or two flare-ups and never encounter symptoms again, while others experience regular flare-ups.

There are the three main types of JRA:

- **Pauciarticular**-onset JRA tends to affect four or less joints. This is the most common variation, accounting for about 50 per cent of cases. It usually affects the large joints such as the knees and occurs more frequently in girls than in boys. As serious eye problems such as inflammation of the iris can also arise, regular ophthalmologist visits are essential. It is common for a child with pauciaticular arthritis to outgrow the condition by adulthood. Eye problems can continue, however, and sometimes joint problems can return.
- **Polyarticular**-onset JRA tends to affect five or more joints. This type accounts for about 30 per cent of cases and again is more common in girls than in boys. It is usual for the small joints in the hands and feet to be attacked by this type of arthritis, but the larger joints can also be involved. In most cases, the condition is symmetrical, affecting the same joint on both sides of the body. Some children with polyarticular arthritis have a particular antibody in their blood called IgM rheumatoid factor. This causes the condition to be more severe, similar to adult RA.
- **Systemic**-onset JRA (also known as Still's disease) causes marked feverishness and a light pink rash. This type accounts for about 20 per cent of cases and both sexes are affected equally. Internal organs such as the heart, liver, spleen and lymph nodes are affected and, very occasionally, the lungs as well. A small number of children with systemic onset juvenile arthritis develop severe arthritis in many joints, continuing into adulthood.

What causes JRA?

As with adult RA, JRA is an auto-immune condition. This means that the body mistakenly identifies some of its own tissues and cells as foreign bodies and sets up an attack on them. The result of this is inflammation, which causes heat, redness, pain and swelling. Scientists suspect that, as with adult RA, a genetic defect causes a predisposition to developing JRA. It may then be triggered off by a virus, infection, injury, environmental factors or something else that is so far unknown.

Researchers are currently attempting to improve existing treatments for all forms of juvenile arthritis. They are also trying to develop more effective drugs – ones that work better and with fewer side effects.

Getting a diagnosis

If your child is experiencing persistent joint pain and swelling, tiredness, unexplained fever and skin rashes and/or swelling of the lymph nodes, he or she should be taken to the doctor. Diagnosis will not be given until the child has been carefully examined, his or her medical history reviewed, and laboratory test results returned. As joint pain and swelling must have been present for at least six months for a diagnosis of JRA to be given, it is important to note when problems first began. For instance, one of the earliest indications of JRA is the child limping slightly in the morning, shortly after getting up. Keep a record of when symptoms first appeared, how they manifest themselves, and when they are worse or better.

Laboratory tests may show that the rheumatoid factor is raised, which helps to confirm a diagnosis of RA. However, these tests are also important for ruling out other conditions such as lupus, bacterial infection, Lyme disease and inflammatory bowel disease. X-rays or an MRI scan may be done if injury to a joint or unusual bone development is suspected.

Treatment

As there is no cure for JRA or any other form of juvenile arthritis, the main aim of treatment is to retain a good level of physical activity and social function. Therefore, it is important to actively treat the swelling, prescribe painkilling drugs and refer the youngster to a physiotherapist in order to maintain a full range of movement in the joints. Some of the drugs recommended for adult RA may also be given to children, but in smaller doses. Your doctor will speak to you about this.

Helping your child to live a happy life in spite of JRA

As well as ensuring that your son or daughter receives good medical care and follows doctor's instructions, parents of children with arthritis should encourage them to do the following:

- attend physiotherapy sessions;
- carry out regular exercise and activity to help keep joints strong and mobile (swimming is particularly beneficial as it exercises many joints and muscles without straining the joints);
- during a remission of symptoms, to take part in team sports; social interaction such as this promotes confidence as well as strength and mobility;
- during a flare-up, to limit their activities, depending upon the areas of the body affected. It is important that children with JRA return to being active as soon as the flare-up is over.

In addition:

- If your child is absent from school for long periods, ask the teachers to send you home assignments and so on.
- Impress on your son or daughter that the condition is not his or her fault in any way and that it can (and does) happen to anyone.
- If the prescribed medications don't work, or cause unpleasant side effects, speak to your doctor about alternatives.

See pages 72–4 for more help for children with arthritis.

Fibromyalgia

Fibromyalgia is an arthritic condition that causes widespread soft tissue pain – that is, in the muscles, tendons and ligaments. It affects between 2 and 4 per cent of the population, is seven times more common in women than in men, and those who get it are usually between the ages of 30 and 60. That said, it can actually develop in any age group, including children and the elderly.

There is, as yet, no cure for fibromyalgia, and the symptoms can fluctuate, sometimes with long periods of remission.

Unlike osteoarthritis and RA, fibromyalgia is not a degenerative condition. In fact, many people gradually improve, so long as they make the recommended lifestyle adjustments (eating healthily, following a regular exercise regime, positive planning, pacing themselves, avoiding stress and so on). On the other hand, inactivity, stress, a poor diet and a negative mindset can provoke numerous flare-ups and so hinder the body's natural instinct to repair itself (and go into remission).

Those who have fibromyalgia often say they 'hurt all over' – although most people hurt more in an area they have used. For instance, after writing for a few hours, the pain may be worse in your neck and shoulders; after cleaning windows, the pain may be worse in one shoulder; or, after walking up the stairs, the discomfort may be worse in your legs. The pain can feel like aching, burning or sharp stabbing.

Fibromyalgia is actually a syndrome, which means that several other conditions are linked to it. These include fatigue, sleep problems, morning stiffness, cognitive problems (known as 'fibro fog'), headaches, irritable bowel syndrome, irritable bladder, anxiety, depression, dry eyes and mouth, numbness and tingling, temperomandibular joint dysfunction (jaw pain), and sensitivity to light, noise, certain chemicals and particular foods and drinks.

After the pain, the fatigue of fibromyalgia is usually the second most prominent symptom. It can range from mild tiredness, to extreme exhaustion that is not dissimilar to that experienced with flu. Sometimes you can feel exhausted before you even get out of bed, yet at other times you may not feel too tired until you have spent a couple of hours walking around the shops.

The sensitivity of fibromyalgia means that even the slightest touch can cause severe pain, lasting for several minutes. If you accidentally hurt yourself – by stubbing your toe for example – the immediate pain can last a good deal longer than it would in someone who doesn't have fibromyalgia. Also, people with the condition have several 'tender points' on their bodies. If, for example, an itch in that site is so much as lightly scratched, the result can be sharp and lingering pain.

Abnormalities in fibromyalgia

There are abnormalities in the following bodily systems in fibromyalgia:

The central nervous system (i.e. the brain and spinal cord)

Advanced scanning technology has shown that people with fibromyalgia have reduced blood flow and energy production in the regions of the brain dealing with pain regulation, memory and concentration. Moreover, neurotransmitters (chemicals that transfer messages from one nerve fibre to another) are unable to properly process pain messages from the central nervous system to other parts of the body. This makes the brain more sensitive to any pain messages it receives and is one reason why there is often constant pain and extreme sensitivity. Another reason for the high levels of pain in fibromyalgia is the greatly elevated levels of a chemical neurotransmitter called substance P. Other conditions involving pain have slight elevations of substance P, but the levels are not nearly so high as in fibromyalgia.

The endocrine system (i.e. the hormones)

Research into the endocrine system has shown that hormonal imbalances play a leading role in fibromyalgia. For instance, there are very low levels of the hormone serotonin, which helps to regulate mood, reduce pain levels, ease muscle tension and helps us to sleep. People with normal levels of serotonin are generally not disposed to mood swings (there are exceptions, of course), they have less pain and muscle tension, and are usually able to sleep better.

The immune system (i.e. antibody protection against infection)

In fibromyalgia, the immune system is disturbed. This is believed to result either from an overload of environmental toxins (e.g. pesticides, aerosols, car fumes) or a viral infection.

Triggering factors

The symptoms of fibromyalgia are usually triggered into action by a particular event, including injury (whiplash injury is a common cause, and was the main trigger in the onset of my own condition), prolonged stress and a viral infection. As the condition often runs in families, it is thought that genetics also play a part. Any defective genes have yet to be discovered, however.

Getting a diagnosis

If you suspect you have fibromyalgia, you should go to your doctor and report your symptoms – writing them down beforehand as a prompt if you think you need to. As yet, there are no simple X-rays, blood tests or scans to diagnose fibromyalgia. You may be referred for tests, though, to rule out other conditions.

The official criteria for diagnosing fibromyalgia are:

- the presence of widespread pain for longer than three months on both sides of the body, above and below the waist;
- pain in at least 11 of the 18 'tender point' sites when they are pressed (see the cartoon below).

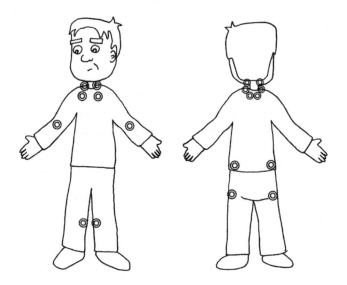

Treating fibromyalgia

As the symptoms of fibromyalgia vary a great deal from person to person, there is no one set treatment regime that fits all. The best results are obtained from using a combination of medications (see below), complementary therapies, lifestyle changes and exercise. The lifestyle changes include pacing, positive thinking, being assertive and learning how to relax, as discussed in my book *Living with Fibromyalgia* (Sheldon Press, 2010).

Some people find that paracetamol gives sufficient pain relief. However, if this drug is not strong enough on its own, you may also be prescribed a tricyclic antidepressant which works by increasing the levels of certain chemicals in the blood. One of these chemicals – serotonin – has already been mentioned (see page 28). Among other things, serotonin helps to reduce pain and improve sleep.

Non-steroidal anti-inflammatory drugs (NSAIDs) (see pages 16–17) are sometimes offered to people with fibromyalgia, particularly during flare-ups. Note, though, that as fibromyalgia is not ordinarily an inflammatory condition, NSAIDs are not usually of benefit. My own fibromyalgia, however, came with a great deal of inflammation, which made my whole spine swollen, hot and extremely painful. Luckily, with the help of NSAIDs and a great deal of self-help, those difficult days are most definitely behind me.

Gout

An attack of gout – an acute form of arthritis – comes on suddenly and swiftly, causing swelling and severe pain in one or more of the joints. Although the base of the big toe is the most common area affected, the condition can affect any joint in the body, as shown in the cartoon opposite.

Men are ten times more at risk of developing gout than women, and it is caused by raised levels of a chemical called 'uric acid' (or 'urate') – a type of waste material that travels around the body in the clear part of the blood, which is known as plasma.

We all have uric acid in our blood, but gout can develop:

• if your body makes too much uric acid;

OR:

• if your kidneys fail to eliminate it quickly enough, as a result of poor kidney function or kidney disease.

It looks like I've been frolicking
in a field of arrows!

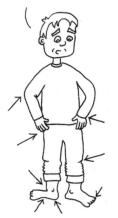

When levels of uric acid are too high, tiny crystals can collect in the tissues – particularly around the joints – causing the swelling and pain of gout. The affected joint will feel hot, the skin will be red and shiny and, if you have had gout on and off for several years, there may even be firm white lumps beneath the skin called 'tophi'. During an attack, many people feel generally unwell and have a slight fever.

When is gout likely to develop?

The following factors can increase your likelihood of developing gout:

- drinking excess alcohol
- being overweight
- having high blood pressure
- having a family history of gout
- consuming a lot of foods containing purines, which are broken down into uric acid (purines are present in red meat, offal, seafood, asparagus, beans, cauliflower, lentils, mushrooms, oatmeal and spinach)
- taking medications such as diuretics that increase the flow of urine from the body

- getting an injury to a joint – for example, gout can be triggered by a knock to the big toe.

A person who is prone to experiencing attacks of gout should try to identify and avoid the things that trigger them. Repeated flare-ups of gout can result in complications – for example, the condition spreading to other joints, tophi appearing, kidney stones forming, and eventual kidney damage.

Getting a diagnosis

Assuming that you go to see your doctor when a joint first becomes swollen, red and very painful, the area affected will be carefully examined. If your doctor suspects gout, a sample of your blood is likely to be tested in a laboratory to measure the levels of uric acid present.

It is important that you remind your doctor of any medications you take, any other illnesses you have, and whether you injured the area before the flare-up occurred.

Treating gout

If the diagnosis is gout, you can reduce the pain and swelling of a flare-up by raising and resting the affected limb – on a stool, perhaps. You should also keep the joint cool by applying an ice pack or bag of frozen peas wrapped in a thin cloth for about

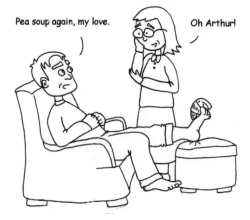

twenty minutes (applying ice directly to the skin can damage it). Allow the area to return to normal temperature before re-administering the treatment.

Where medicines are concerned, you may find that para-cetamol reduces pain sufficiently to get you through an attack. Paracetamol is not always adequate, however, in which case you may be offered NSAIDs to tackle the pain and inflammation. There is also a drug family called **colchicines** which work by reducing the build-up of uric acid. Side effects are a problem for some who take colchicines, though, as they can induce nausea, vomiting and diarrhoea. If you encounter such problems when taking these drugs, you should see your doctor – there may be an alternative in the colchicines family with fewer side effects, or you may be able to lower the initial dose and build up gradually.

A person who experiences repeated attacks of gout is likely to be offered a medicine called **allopurinol**. When taken daily, this drug increases the volume of uric acid removed from the kidneys.

You can also help yourself by losing excess weight, eating a healthy low-purine diet, having only a small amount of alcohol, and drinking up to 2 litres of water a day. It is also important to identify and avoid triggering factors, as mentioned above. (See page 43 for information about cherries, which have been found to be excellent in reducing the pain and inflammation of gout flare-ups.)

2

Natural remedies

Medication undoubtedly has its place in the treatment of arthritis. It can be invaluable, for example, in getting you through a flare-up of symptoms and helping you to sleep. In some cases, drugs can even assist in halting the progression of the condition. However, many experts believe that the use of natural remedies is equally important, if not more so – and that many people would be best advised to manage the condition with the help of natural remedies in conjunction with drugs.

It should be said that there are those who are able to manage their arthritis with the use of natural remedies and other self-help measures alone, which is terrific as it greatly reduces the amount of chemicals in the body. Whether you can be one of these people will depend on the severity of your arthritis, your ability to find natural remedies and treatments that work well for you, and your persistence in following a self-help regime.

Before taking natural remedies, please heed the following:

- Be aware that no natural remedy can *cure* arthritis, whether it is advertised as doing so or not. Really what you should be aiming for is symptom management in the form of less pain, improved mobility and so on.
- Before taking a particular remedy, find out as much as you can about it.
- Speak to your doctor to check whether a particular remedy could interact with your prescription drugs.
- When taking a remedy, keep a record of how you feel so you can tell whether it is working.
- Only purchase brands from reputable companies. (See the Useful addresses section at the back of this book for details of two trustworthy outlets.)

When to use natural remedies

Many people swear by natural remedies such as cider vinegar, barley grass juice, noni juice and other products. So do they really work? In the following pages I try to base my opinion concerning each remedy on scientific facts rather than anecdotal endorsements (in the form of unproven testimonials, and so on). The more conventional herbal and vitamin remedies such as glucosamine, chondroitin and devil's claw are acclaimed by millions of people with arthritis, and are explored later in this chapter.

Please note, though, that it isn't a case of 'one size fits all'. Indeed, what provides relief for one person may actually worsen symptoms for someone else. It is important, therefore, to try out a few remedies – preferably those that are recommended for treating arthritis – before deciding which works best for you.

Apple cider vinegar

Unprocessed apple cider vinegar is seen by many as a miraculous tonic containing a powerful combination of healing properties. Beta carotene is believed to be one of those properties, its chief function in the body being to destroy the harmful molecules – known as 'free radicals' – that are involved in ageing, mutation of tissues and destruction of the immune system. People who advocate the use of apple cider vinegar claim that it contains dozens of beneficial components that have an anti-ageing effect, preventing germs, parasites and infectious diseases from invading the body and combating a variety of ailments such as chronic fatigue, diabetes, digestive problems and migraines. It is also claimed to help reduce high blood pressure and high cholesterol.

Perhaps apple cider vinegar is best known, though, as a curative for arthritis. Exponents of it have long made the assumption that, in arthritis, acid crystals form in the joints and tissues, resulting in the stiff joints and hardened tissues that characterize the condition. They believe that apple cider vinegar dissolves these harmful crystals so they can be flushed from the body in the urine, effectively stopping the progression of arthritis and encouraging the body to heal itself. There is no denying the great bulk of anecdotal recommendations supporting this belief. Indeed, lots of people with arthritis profess to have benefited greatly from a daily intake of apple cider vinegar, and some claim complete recovery as a result.

You may be interested to learn, however, that there is now a growing body of experts who strongly oppose the notion that apple cider vinegar has medicinal properties. They state that there is absolutely no scientific evidence to back up the anecdotal claims and that apple cider vinegar is anything but a storehouse of nutrients. Taking one to two teaspoonfuls of apple cider vinegar (with honey) two to three times a day is recommended by its advocates, yet when one tablespoonful underwent laboratory analysis, less than one gram of carbohydrate and only miniscule amounts of calcium, iron, magnesium, sodium, manganese, potassium and phosphorus were found. Moreover, it contained no fibre, no vitamins and no amino acids. Scientists believe the lack of beneficial enzymes is due to their being unable to survive the acid environment of vinegar – and if they did by some miracle happen to survive it, they would quickly be destroyed by the acid in our stomachs.

In 1985, an Alabama farmer called Jack McWilliams combined apple cider vinegar with fruit juices to improve the taste. He believed today's diet is far too low in acetic acid and that this deficiency is the root of many health problems. Calling his potion 'Jogging in a Jug', he asserted that it could cure arthritis and heart disease and reduce the risk of cancer. Mr McWilliams is reported to have sold nine million dollars' worth of his product in one year – however, the US Food and Drug Administration (FDA) were sceptical of the product and, in 1994, seized and destroyed thousands of bottles, citing unproven health claims as the reason. Mr McWilliams was ordered to pay a large fine to settle charges of false advertising. 'Jogging in a Jug' is back on the market, but the advertising is now modest with no unproven claims.

Although the arthritis associations I contacted declined to offer their opinions on apple cider vinegar, the Arthritis Foundation refers to it on their website as 'a harmless, but unproven, arthritis remedy'. It stresses that arthritis symptoms commonly come and go and that if an unproven remedy were used at a time when symptoms were in decline, it would be easy to think that the remedy had worked. The Foundation states its belief that this is clearly what has happened for many who use vinegar-related remedies.

Having said that, if you are taking apple cider vinegar and believe you are better for doing so, it is recommended that you continue the regime. If something works for you, it works – regardless of whether the science backs it up or experts believe the improvement coincides with a remission. I tried taking apple cider vinegar myself recently, but was forced to stop after a few days as it was clearly worsening the inflammation (arthritis) in my neck and provoking more muscle pain than ever (that is, worsening my fibromyalgia). A friend with RA had a similar reaction. Some people experience digestive problems when using apple cider vinegar, and so have no choice but to cease taking it.

It's impossible, though, to ignore the thousands of people who swear by this product, so I would suggest that it's worth a tentative try. According to proponents of this regime, the best apple cider vinegar is ruddy in colour with a discernible amount of residue floating around in the bottle. One to three teaspoonfuls should be mixed into 8 ounces of water three times daily and taken before meals. Honey can be mixed into the drink to make it more palatable.

Barley grass juice

Barley grass has been cultivated for thousands of years and is still used as a cereal food source in parts of Asia. People the world over have long used barley grass juice as a tonic and natural energy source – however, it wasn't until the start of the twentieth century that it was subjected to a great deal of scientific research and found to be an excellent source of nutrients required by the body for growth, repair and wellbeing. Its attributes are in no small part due to the presence of an important substance called P4D1, which has strong anti-inflammatory properties and has been shown in laboratory testing to actually repair human DNA (DNA being a carrier of genetic material that occurs in every cell in the body). Damaged DNA leads to ageing, disease and eventual death. Where arthritis is concerned, the high sodium content and anti-inflammatory properties of barley grass help to slow down the progression of the condition. Indeed, many of those with arthritis using this juice have experienced significant pain relief within a week or two.

Many experts are of the opinion that barley grass has the most balanced nutrient profile of all green plants and that these nutrients work together as powerful antioxidants to protect our bodies from damage from free radicals. The particular combination of nutrients in barley grass is also believed to boost immune system function and improve cardiovascular health.

Dr Howard Lutz, director of the Institute of Preventative Medicine in Washington DC, says that barley grass is one of the most incredible products of our era. He adds that it improves stamina, sexual energy, clarity of thought and reduces addictive impulses. He says also that barley grass juice improves the skin texture and heals the dryness associated with ageing.

Horses and cows, with their elongated digestive tracts, are able to break down the indigestible cellulose fibres of barley grass and therefore release its nutrients. Unfortunately, we humans have less efficient digestive systems that are unable to break down either cellulose or fibre. We can not, therefore, obtain the nutrients in barley grass simply by eating it. In fact, barley grass is more easily digestible in juice form, and it should only be consumed in that way. Grasses that are sown in early spring and late autumn on certified organic farms are said to be the most beneficial to health. The grass is washed, 'juiced', and dried at cold temperatures before the resultant powder is hermetically sealed into vacuum-packed bags. Barley grass powders that have been cultured in greenhouse trays or processed in a different way are said to have minimal health benefits.

I recently attended a discussion on the benefits of barley grass juice given by the owner of a major grass juicing company. I was impressed by his knowledge and interested in the first-hand accounts of the many different ways in which the juice was helping those present. These people included friends of mine, and I had actually noticed an improvement in their appearance, without knowing the reason. I was handed a glass of bright green juice and found that it tasted rather as expected – like grass! It wasn't actually unpleasant – more an 'acquired taste'. I suspect that as the news spreads regarding the benefits of barley grass juice, it will become a chief constituent of natural therapy. Please see the Useful addresses section for details of where you can purchase good-quality barley grass juice products. It certainly won't put me off giving barley grass juice a good try over the next few months. After only two weeks of taking it, I feel more energized and have found that my hair is shinier, my nails are stronger, and my skin is less dry. I'm already very pleased and hope for more improvements as time goes by.

Noni juice

Noni juice is derived from the fruit of the *Morinda citrifolia* tree which commonly flourishes in Polynesia, but that is most prevalent on the Pacific island of Tahiti. The juice is therefore often termed 'Tahitian noni'.

The pungent odour of the fruit when ripening has earned it the informal name of 'vomit fruit'. Its taste is very bitter, too, yet it remains a common food on some Pacific islands. The pulp, bark, leaves and seeds of the noni fruit have been used as a healing tonic for inflammation, constipation, respiratory problems and other conditions for over 2,000 years. More recently, the juice of the fruit has been mixed with more palatable fruit flavours and marketed in the West as 'a miracle in a bottle'. As a consequence, the manufacture of noni juice is a multi-million-dollar industry with a loyal following who swear by its health benefits – though there are many inconsistencies in the testimonials of those who use it. It is even said that the Polynesians themselves only resorted to taking the juice as a health tonic when all other avenues had failed.

There is no doubt that noni fruit powder is rich in carbohydrates, fibre and other beneficial health-giving agents. However, when the juice of the noni fruit was analysed in a laboratory, a surprisingly small quantity of these nutrients were detected. Indeed, one medicinal helping of noni juice was found to contain no more health-giving properties than are present in one orange. Scientists concluded, therefore, that the high nutrient content of noni is stored in the pulp of the fruit rather than in the juice.

In 2007, a large noni juice manufacturer hired actor Danny Glover to promote the health benefits of the juice. The advertising campaign was successful and many people purchased the juice in the hope of improving their health. But after the spotlight was thrown on noni juice in a CBS news investigation and its benefits revealed to be questionable, Mr Glover withdrew his support. Around the same time, immunologist Dr Jeffrey Galpin reviewed noni juice studies (all backed by noni juice manufacturers) and made it clear that the claims of the manufacturers could not be verified. 'It's promoted to do everything with no validation of anything,' he said. However, one of the noni juice distributors by the name of Jeanette Bush insists that the juice has performed miracles and that the company she works for is not selling false hope to people in need. It can't be ignored, though, that in 1998 the manufacturers of noni juice were charged by the Attorneys General of several US states with making unfounded health claims. They were ordered to stop advertising the purported benefits until scientific back-up could be provided. This has not happened but the juice continues to be advertised in other US states.

I should mention here that France has warned prospective purchasers of the risks of noni juice, saying that severe liver problems were found in some after drinking the juice. It should therefore not be used by people with liver problems. Diabetics, too, should monitor their noni intake very carefully as it is high in sugar. Constipation is a common side effect of noni juice, particularly if high amounts are consumed. A further possible side effect is coughing and wheezing. If you still wish to try noni juice, it is recommended that you visit your doctor before starting it. You should build up intake very gradually, monitoring the effect very carefully.

Clearly, much more research is required into the possible health benefits (and dangers) of the product. It is to be hoped that this takes place.

Aloe vera juice

The aloe vera plant has a long history as a folk remedy and is known all over the world as the 'first aid plant' or 'medicine plant'. Both gel and latex can be extracted from the plant, the

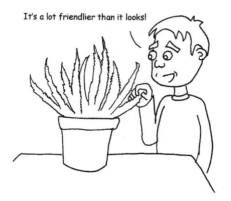

It's a lot friendlier than it looks!

gel being clear, jelly-like pulp from the inner part of the leaves and the latex being a bitter yellow substance that is carried in tiny tubes beneath the outer skin of the leaves. It is the latex that is commonly known as 'aloe juice' and that is now widely used to treat a variety of conditions, including arthritis and digestive tract problems.

After conducting several studies into the properties of aloe juice, scientists concluded that because it is packed with a particular combination of nutrients – inclusive of vitamins, minerals and amino acids – it is capable of relieving the pain of arthritis. Aloe juice was also found to be high in 'basic sugars' (known as mucopolysaccharides), which are normally present in every cell in the body and need replenishment on a regular basis. All these substances, in combination, are thought to make aloe juice an immune-system stimulant, a powerful anti-inflammatory, and a good analgesic (painkiller). It is also believed that aloe juice can prevent further damage and speed up cell repair, which should effectively alleviate pain and help to dislodge damaged tissue for elimination via the urine.

Numerous studies worldwide have been carried out into the effects of aloe juice, and it would appear to be capable of improving a wide range of medical conditions. Strangely, though, I could find little direct research into the effects of this product on arthritis. After looking at websites that display comments from those with arthritis, it became clear to me that the success of aloe juice treatment varies considerably from person to person. Some individuals report dramatic pain relief and improved joint mobility, whereas others say they waited a long time for any improvements and in the end there was little or no change. Which people are likely to respond best cannot be predicted and I can only assume that this therapy is more successful if used in the early stages of arthritis and perhaps in those who don't smoke and are successful in making positive lifestyle changes, as discussed in this book.

The side effects of taking aloe juice seem to be rare, with the exception of pink-coloured urine. In a small number of people it can apparently cause electrolyte loss, fluid imbalance, intestinal cramps and slow healing of wounds, but only if the person overdoses or takes fairly large quantities of the product for a lengthy period. Side effects don't normally occur if you follow the label instructions on the bottle.

Aloe juice and its effects on arthritis is another area in which further research would be welcome and we can only hope that it takes place soon. In the meantime, taking aloe juice can apparently do no harm, and may even be of substantial benefit.

Emu oil

Emu oil is a natural remedy that has been used in Australian Aboriginal medicine for hundreds of years. However, it is now becoming famous worldwide as a soothing agent for a variety of health problems. Where arthritis is concerned, its apparent ability to reduce inflammation, stiffness and pain when externally applied to the area affected recently brought it to the attention of researchers, and several scientifically controlled studies have now been carried out. In all such studies, a reduction in symptoms was seen, with scientists stating that in some cases the topical application of emu oil was more effective than non-steroidal anti-inflammatory drugs (NSAIDs) such as ibuprofen, but without the risk of side effects. Some studies showed a better outcome than others – but scientists suspect the disparity was caused by the quality of the oil (some companies seemingly produce superior oil than others).

Dr P. Ghoosh, an Australian research scientist and international authority on osteoarthritis, asserts that laboratory experiments have consistently confirmed the therapeutic value of emu oil for people with arthritis. He even claims that it offers the very best relief available for the condition.

Emu oil comes in pure oil form or is mixed with other anti-inflammatory herbs to enhance its efficacy. A topical product, it is massaged into the skin where it penetrates quickly and completely, healing and nourishing the skin at cellular level. Researchers claim that, unlike petroleum-based products, emu oil has a fatty acid composition similar to the oil in human skin and it is this that enables it to penetrate the skin, giving pain relief in 15 minutes or less. Emu oil also contains vitamins A and E – antioxidants that fight damage from free radicals. Free radicals are unstable molecules that damage our cells, contributing to ageing and age-related diseases. Dr Leigh Hopkins, a clinical professor of pharmacology, even says that emu oil helps to normalize basic cellular function and allows the body to return to normal healing.

Although I would like to see even more scientific evidence regarding the efficacy of emu oil, I think it is safe to say that it is usually a beneficial treatment for the symptoms of arthritis.

Montmorency cherry juice

Montmorency cherry juice has recently become a popular treatment for inflammatory conditions. Indeed, drinking this type of cherry juice on a daily basis has been shown in ongoing research on animals to reduce the pain and inflammation of arthritis like no other fruit or vegetable. The presence of natural antioxidants and powerful substances called **anthocyanins** (pigments) is what is believed to make montmorency cherry juice so effective. In fact, research has shown that montmorency cherry juice works in the same way as NSAIDs. Unlike NSAIDs, though, this cherry juice seems to offer protection against stomach irritation.

Some researchers claim that montmorency cherry juice is as effective in reducing pain as aspirin and ibuprofen, but without the risk of side effects such as stomach ulcers and kidney damage. It is apparently the antioxidants in these cherries that vastly reduce the risk of side effects. Melatonin – one antioxidant that is present in this type of cherry juice – has been subject to much testing on people with sleep problems, the outcome being that normal sleep patterns usually return when using this substance. Poor sleep is a major contributing factor of fibromyalgia and this can be helped greatly by taking montmorency cherry juice on a regular basis.

Although I don't doubt that the juice is a good natural replacement for anti-inflammatory drugs, I would like to see it undergo more scientifically controlled studies. There have been some very promising research studies on rats with arthritis where the **cyanidin** in cherries was seen to protect against paw inflammation and where antioxidant activity was improved, but we need to see this effect in a series of human studies.

I can testify that drinking montmorency cherry juice is a wonderfully pleasant form of self-medication. Montmorency cherries are available in juice concentrate; they can also be freeze-dried into powder that is placed in capsules. (See the Useful addresses section at the back of this book for details of where to purchase this product.)

Other natural remedies

Many people with arthritis use natural remedies such as glucosamine, chondroitin and so on. In this section I look at whether or not these substances do what they are supposed to do, and examine whether they are safe.

Glucosamine and chondroitin

Glucosamine hydrochloride is an amino sugar that occurs naturally in high concentrations in all the joints of the human body. It is even believed to be involved in the formation and repair of cartilage. **Chondroitin sulphate**, a carbohydrate, is actually a main component of cartilage, giving cartilage resilience and impeding the enzymes that break it down. Glucosamine and chondroitin have been used together as a combination therapy for several years.

Many people with arthritis – particularly osteoarthritis – take glucosamine and chondroitin on a daily basis and some speak of their benefits in glowing terms. There have even been research studies that strongly suggest these nutrients can relieve the stiffness and pain of arthritis (especially in the knees), and with fewer side effects than found with conventional arthritis drugs. Please note that glucosamine and chondroitin do not *cure* arthritis, despite the way in which they are sometimes advertised. In fact, after people in a number of recent studies reported no improvements at all, the efficacy of glucosamine and chondroitin was thrown into doubt. Finally, an expert review body was set up to look at the available evidence and concluded that more scientifically controlled studies are required. The main reason for this is that although most studies had a positive outcome, those with a negative outcome were larger and far better designed. They were clearly more reliable, therefore.

To date, the largest and best-designed clinical trial[2] involved 1,583 volunteers with arthritis of the knee. During a 24-week period in 2006 they were randomly given either glucosamine, chondroitin (see below), celecoxib (a prescription drug, see page 18) or a placebo (simple sugar pill) three times daily. The conclusion was that glucosamine and chondroitin, taken alone or together, did not reduce symptoms more effectively than a placebo in those with mild to moderate pain. Those with severe pain showed a very slight improvement, and the ones taking celecoxib reported a significant (17 per cent) improvement.

The studies that showed a positive outcome – indicating that glucosamine and/or chondroitin are more effective than a placebo in relieving symptoms – generally lasted for only about four weeks, were less rigid, and had a much smaller number of volunteers in the trials. Clearly, there is a need for larger, more rigidly controlled studies into these two nutrients. In the meantime, if you decide to try them you should look for improvements within two months. If you have already taken this combination remedy for over two months and your pain is no better, it is advisable that you stop. The large study mentioned above suggested that only people with *severe* arthritis in the knee will respond to glucosamine and chondroitin therapy.

Glucosamine is not specifically recommended by the NHS as being helpful in arthritis.

Fish oils

There is much anecdotal evidence that fish oils, such as cod liver oil, can bring about a moderate improvement in the joint stiffness and pain of arthritis. However, why fish oil is apparently so helpful was not known until October 2009, when it was discovered that the body converts the omega 3 essential fatty acids (EFAs) in fish oils into a powerful anti-inflammatory chemical known as **resolvin D2**.

Scientists are now hoping that resolvin D2 will provide the basis for a range of important new treatments for inflammatory conditions.

Omega 3 is obtained from oily fish such as mackerel, sardines, herring, tuna, etc., vegetable oils, seeds (sunflower seeds, sesame seeds, linseeds (sometimes known as flaxseed), etc.), nuts and avocados. Oils should be stored in a sealed container in a cool, dark place to prevent rancidity.

All oils are a natural source of vitamin E, which is an important antioxidant. Antioxidants are essential to cell life because they mop up the destructive 'free radicals' within the body. Unfortunately, when food is processed in some way (this means when it is prepared or converted by being boiled, for example, and/or having other substances added), the vitamin E in some unsaturated oils is removed, depriving the body of its benefits. Processed oils are also susceptible to rancidity. It is recommended, therefore, that you obtain your fats from natural sources (see the above paragraph). If you don't think you obtain sufficient essential fatty acids from your diet, you may wish to try supplementation in the form of fish oil capsules. Follow the instructions on the label and take the oil for at least three to six months to get the full effects. Any benefit is lost when you stop the fish oil supplements.

See page 96 for more information on omega 3 versus omega 6 EFAs.

Evening primrose oil

Although this herbal supplement has long been known as an immune system regulator, trials aimed at proving or disproving this claim have been inconclusive. Note that evening primrose oil may be detrimental to those with overactive immune systems, as occurs in RA and lupus, and they are advised to steer clear of it.

If you think it is safe for you to try evening primrose oil, keep in mind that it takes three to six months for the full benefits to be apparent. Any improvement is lost when you stop taking it.

MSM (methyl sulfonyl methane)

Some people claim that MSM is a cure for arthritis, but there is no scientific evidence either to back this up or prove its safety. MSM is present in fresh foods such as fruit and vegetables, dairy products, fish and grains. Food that is not fresh – that is, it has undergone processing in some form – loses its MSM content.

This compound is available in capsules and as a lotion.

SAMe (S-adenosylmethionine)

A range of studies have shown that this supplement can boost levels of certain amino acids, improving joint mobility, easing pain and reducing inflammation. Indeed, it is claimed that SAMe can alleviate pain to the same degree as NSAIDs. Nausea and an upset stomach are possible side effects, however.

Cat's claw

Extracted from a Peruvian vine, cat's claw is widely used in South America for treating joint inflammation and pain. To date, there has been no research on its effects in humans, but studies with animals have shown that it can act as an antioxidant and anti-inflammatory. It is available in capsules, as well as in teabags so you can drink it, and you should be careful to select the *Uncaria tomentosa* variety as other types can be toxic. Note that cat's claw can increase the risk of bleeding if taken with blood thinners such as warfarin or heparin.

Devil's claw

Devil's claw is derived from an African plant, the roots of which are believed to contain anti-inflammatory and painkilling properties. Although it is widely used for treating RA, studies have so far been inconclusive. It is available in the form of capsules and teabags, but because it stimulates stomach acid it should not be used if you have digestive problems and/or a stomach ulcer. Ensure that the product you buy contains *harpagoside*, the active ingredient.

Cayenne

Also called capsaicin, cayenne is made from ground chillies and, when applied externally as a cream, is said to temporarily ease the pain of arthritis. Chillies trigger the release of endorphins – the body's natural painkillers; they also interfere with a chemical responsible for sending pain signals – and can therefore block pain for a time. You should only apply cayenne cream to unbroken skin and you must thoroughly wash your hands after using it.

Ginger

Research has shown that ginger root can inhibit the production of the chemicals involved in inflammation and pain – it therefore shows great potential. It can be used in generous amounts in cooking and to flavour herbal teas. It also comes in tablet and powder form.

Beware, however, if you are taking blood-thinning drugs such as warfarin and heparin, as when combined with ginger they can increase the risk of bleeding.

Boswellia

Also known as frankincense, boswellia comes from an Asian gum tree. It has been used for many years in Indian ayurvedic medicine to treat the inflammation in arthritis, as well as the muscular pains that come with conditions such as fibromyalgia. However, the results of studies into its efficacy have been inconclusive and there is a need for better-quality trials. If you experience diarrhoea, a rash or nausea, it is best to stop taking it.

Green tea

Green tea contains compounds called **phenols** which work as antioxidants in alleviating pain and reducing inflammation. Studies in animals have shown that it could be useful for treating RA in particular, but of course human research studies are needed. Note that you shouldn't add milk to your cup of green tea as this could render the phenols useless. As well as being available in teabags, green tea comes in tablet or capsule form.

3

Helping yourself on a practical level

In order to manage your arthritis and so get more out of life, you would be best advised to make a few positive lifestyle changes. Some of these suggestions are discussed in further chapters, but in this chapter I would like to tackle such things as 'pacing' and 'listening to your body'.

Doing this can:

- reduce pain and inflammation;
- improve your mobility and range of motion;
- boost your energy levels;
- improve your physical strength;
- (possibly) reduce the amount of medication you need to take;
- give you better rest and sleep;
- reduce your stress levels.

How to use 'pacing'

'Pacing' is an energy and lifestyle management strategy through which the rhythm of over-activity followed by set-backs – as usually occurs in arthritis – can be avoided, enabling symptoms to become more stable. It involves not overdoing any type of activity, or rest, with the result that in time you will be able to balance activity with appropriate rest periods. Activity and rest periods should always be alternated, with the aim of very gradually increasing activity and reducing rest.

It is important that any activity is split into manageable portions and that, if possible, you switch from one type of activity to another before taking a planned rest. Of course, changing from one activity to another is not always feasible, especially if you need to do something time-consuming such as going to the shops. However, if you can do it at least some of the time, it can prevent an increase in pain.

Note that as very little research has been carried out to show that pacing is effective as a pain- and energy-management technique, there is some controversy about it. That said, anyone who uses it properly will gladly tell you how effective it is.

Planning your everyday life

Individuals with arthritis really need to plan their lives on a day-to-day basis. Living in this way may seem artificial – but it gives back the sense that you are once more in control, which is enormously mood enhancing.

Most people with arthritis are inclined to treat the condition the way they would treat any other illness, by resting when they feel bad – which is invariably after overdoing things. Changing to living a planned life, rather than pushing ahead and then reacting to symptoms as they arise, is often a real challenge, but well worth it if your arthritis gradually becomes more stable.

'Listening to your body'

Some people are not used to tuning into the messages produced by their bodies – but to use the pacing technique with any degree of success you really need to. If you determine to be vigilant in looking out for an increase in symptoms, you will definitely notice them. At the very first sign of increasing discomfort, stop what you are doing and take a relaxing break. If you don't react to the pain, you are likely to find yourself with a flare-up of symptoms and needing more rest than you had bargained for. So, for the sake of stability and slowing down the progression of your arthritis, it is vital that you 'listen' to what your body is 'telling' you.

Rest periods in between activities

When planning your day, remember the need to rest between activities. Obviously, the most demanding of activities require longer rest periods afterwards than the less demanding. Every time you fail to rest sufficiently after a demanding activity, you bring yourself one step closer to a pain flare-up.

Don't forget that it is best to rest only for as long as you think you need to, and no longer. It is also important to alternate activities you find demanding with ones you find more manageable.

Alternate tiring and less tiring activities

It is recommended that you get on with your most demanding activites when you are feeling your best. Saving your most taxing of activities until late on in the day means you have less energy to work with, which will bring on symptoms a lot quicker than if you had tackled the activity earlier on.

Since following a daily exercise routine is of paramount importance, it is also advisable to carry this out early in the day (see Chapter 7 for information on exercise).

When there are several tiring or very tiring activities

If your planned day consists of several activities you find demanding, you need to rearrange your week so that you aren't carrying out more than you can reasonably cope with in one day. You therefore need to think hard about what it is actually essential that you do. The whole idea of pacing is that you not only spread out the more difficult of your tasks, but also that you drop certain activities – with the exception of an exercise regime – until your symptoms decrease.

If you think it is not possible for you to drop even the most demanding of your activities – perhaps because you live alone – remember that there are solutions to virtually everything in life if you have the insight to look for them and the courage to implement them. For example, you might not like asking family and friends to help out, but for the sake of your health and the chance of improvement, it needs to be done. If you can possibly afford a cleaner, I would strongly advise that you employ one. A friend or relative who helps out may even be entitled to claim benefits from the social services, or you yourself may be able to claim. Any benefit you receive is intended as a 'purse' from which you can pay for cleaners, gardeners, taxis, someone to do shopping, and any other help you need. For people who have no one at all to help out, it is vital that you speak to your doctor about help from the social services and occupational therapy departments (see pages 106–7 for more information).

If you live with a partner and have children who are at least eight years old, you really need to ask them for help with the activities you find most taxing. For instance, you could ask your partner to help with housework and either to do the shopping, or accompany you to the shops, so that they can do most of the carrying (if carrying is a problem), and maybe even the driving (if that also is a problem). Note that there is nothing wrong with asking children of eight or over to dry the dishes and do a little dusting, vacuuming and other light duties. Children of 13 and over could be taught how to do the washing and ironing and how to make certain meals – in this way, you are not only helping yourself, you are also preparing your children for adult life. Of course, youngsters are always more willing to help if you remember to thank and praise them, and ensure that they still have plenty of time for themselves. Those under the age of eight should not be expected to do much housework, but can run upstairs to fetch you a jumper, help to whisk the Yorkshire pudding batter, bring you a drink of juice and so on – simple jobs that make them feel useful and that are a great help to you.

When enjoyable activities cause pain

In order to feel a lot better than you are at present, emotional nourishment is just as important as practical matters (emotional help is covered in Chapter 4). If at all possible, therefore, you should try to do at least one activity a day that gives you pleasure. So what do you do about those activities you enjoy but that exacerbate your symptoms?

Caroline
Caroline, 47, loves to embroider cushion covers to sell on an internet auction site. Producing an admired piece of work makes her feel good about herself, as does making money from it. It is therefore important to her that she continues her hobby. She usually embroiders for two hours a day in one session, but recently started to wonder if this was preventing the arthritis in her finger joints from settling down. So she resolved to spend no more than half an hour at a time on it twice daily and to do absolutely no more than that. After a week of this regime, her fingers were already less stiff and painful. In the second week, though, because she was feeling a lot better, she allowed herself to get carried

away and work on one cushion for over an hour. She was faintly aware that the pain in her finger joints was increasing, but in her determination to finish the work she ignored the signals sent out by her body. As a consequence, she had no option but to put her work aside and rest her hands until the pain had subsided once more. For Caroline, this takes several days.

When pain doesn't seem to improve with pacing

Derek
At 66, Derek had already had to give up his daily round of golf, his favourite pastime, due to the pain in his arthritic hip. The pain was increasing so fast that it wasn't a case of doing less so that ultimately he would be able to do more. He can no longer manage to walk to the local shop and so really misses the sense of independence he had. In fact, he is quite depressed and can't wait until the date of his hip replacement surgery.

Derek found that cutting back his golf to every other day didn't really help, even when he rested all morning in anticipation. His arthritis was just too aggressive. He tried playing once a week instead, but his hip joint stiffened so much in the intervening periods that this regime didn't work. So, he resorted to sitting in front of the TV all day, feeling miserable and getting under his wife's feet.

In some people, arthritis progresses so rapidly that the benefits of pacing aren't always apparent. However, the technique is still very important as pushing yourself too far inevitably causes a 'crash' – this is known as the 'push/crash cycle'. And, sadly, those with severe arthritis who overdo things come crashing down more heavily than those with milder arthritis. In effect, then, pacing is *more* important to someone with severe arthritis. It helps the inflammation to calm down, thus decreasing the rate of damage to the affected joints.

If Derek had actually exchanged his game of golf for, say, a daily walk to the local shop less than half a mile away, the inflammation would have been more likely to settle down and a fairly good range of movement maintained in the joint. His condition would then most likely have slowed down and the pain been far less. Derek's other options might have been to take up a different hobby such as playing bowls, joining the nearest gym, swimming or doing aqua-aerobics at his local pool – making sure, of course, not to push himself too far in the new activity.

Unfortunately, for some people the flare-ups keep on coming, no matter how much they avoid overdoing things. Therefore they soon reach the stage where they are spending most of the day resting, afraid to do the slightest thing for fear of it exacerbating the problem. I was at this stage myself during the 1990s, but have since slowly fought my way back to better health. Medication has always had its place in reducing my pain, but it was the other lifestyle changes I made – all of which are discussed in this book – that really made the difference.

Coping with special occasions

You may already be using pacing and other positive lifestyle changes in your daily life and have found that the inflammatory process has largely settled down. Special occasions, though, such as weddings, birthday parties and Christmas celebrations, can threaten your new-found stability, but there are strategies that can help you cope. This means that you don't always have to avoid events you might otherwise have enjoyed.

The enjoyment factor

If the affected joints are still very swollen and painful and you know the event in question would only exacerbate things, don't even think about attending – and certainly don't let yourself be pressurized into it. On the other hand, if your symptoms are stable or starting to stabilize, it is useful to take the enjoyment factor into account. For instance, try asking yourself if this is the type of event you might have enjoyed if you didn't have arthritis, or whether it's an event you would, in the past, have found tedious anyway. If the latter is the case, don't even think about attending – it just isn't worth it at this stage. However, if it's the former but you don't fancy attending the event, try to work out whether you are unnecessarily over-protecting yourself when, with extra rest and so on, you could probably cope with the event and even get pleasure from it. (See pages 68–72 for information on how best to cope with taxing events.)

The fear factor

Perhaps you have reached the stage where the thought of doing something outside of your normal sphere fills you with dread. Sadly, this mindset is not conducive to improvement as the whole idea of pacing (and the other management techniques mentioned in this book) is to gradually extend what you are able to do.

If you often worry that an enjoyable activity could cause a severe symptom flare-up and so you do very little at all, you may need additional help from a cognitive behavioural therapist (this therapy is known as CBT). This type of therapy teaches you a more positive mindset and enables you to make the necessary preparations for coping with taxing events. (I offer help with this in Chapter 4. Page 56, on taking extra rest, should be of benefit too.)

Explain your limitations

I find that I cope better with special occasions if I quietly inform the people around me that I must stick to my limits, adding that pushing myself could cause a relapse. These people are then not surprised or disappointed if I decide to leave early or ask if I can rest on a bed for an hour. They may even schedule, for the other people attending, an activity requiring physical agility for the period when you are taking a rest.

Using cold and heat to relieve pain

The stiffness and pain of arthritis can be relieved very simply by the use of cold and heat. Cold packs, such as a bag of frozen peas or a freezer 'gel pack' (available from some pharmacies), are particularly useful in an acute flare-up where the inflammatory process is in full swing and causing a lot of pain in the affected joint. In effect, it numbs the area and so decreases the heat and swelling (inflammation). Don't forget, though, to wrap hot and cold packs in a towel or thin cloth to prevent damage to your skin.

People with arthritis of the hands and/or feet respond better to cold packs when alternated with heat treatment as a 'contrast therapy'. This entails filling two bowls – one with warm water at 43°C (110°F) and the other with cold water at 21°C (65°F). Immerse your hands or feet for ten minutes in the cold water, then for ten minutes in the warm water. Repeat the process for as long as you think you need to. Carrying out this treatment at least three times a day during a flare-up can make a great difference and help symptoms to settle down.

There are several types of heat treatment:

- microwaveable heat packs/wheat bags which can be warmed up and placed on a painful area of the body;
- gel packs that can be warmed by immersion in hot water;
- soaking in a warm bath, shower or Jacuzzi;
- dipping stiff painful fingers in a paraffin bath – i.e., a mixture of warm melted paraffin and mineral oil.

Rest and sleep

Getting a good night's sleep is of great importance to all of us. It helps restore our energy levels, gives our joints and soft tissues a chance to rest, and helps us cope with the stress and problems that arise in daily life. Unfortunately, for people with arthritis, a good night's sleep can be elusive.

It is possible to develop good sleep habits by doing the following:

- Take fewer naps, and sleep for a shorter time – no longer than half an hour. All naps can stop you from feeling sleepy at bedtime.
- Hang heavy curtains to make the bedroom as dark as possible.
- Before trying to sleep, unwind by listening to calming music or a relaxation tape or CD, reading, or watching an unexciting programme on TV.
- Have a warm drink.
- Shortly before bedtime, take a hot bath.
- Go to bed when you feel sleepy, but not before 9.30 p.m.
- Ensure that your bed and bedroom are comfortably warm, but not over-heated.
- Wear a sleep mask to sleep soundly for longer periods of time.
- Wear earplugs to eliminate distracting noises.
- Make yourself comfortable in bed, breathing slowly and evenly from your diaphragm. Clear your mind and allow

your thoughts to drift. Don't hold on to any one thought, but let them drift along unchecked.

- Set your alarm for the same time every morning.

Try to avoid the following:

- caffeinated drinks after 6 p.m.;
- alcohol before bedtime;
- engaging in animated conversation (or arguments) just before bedtime;
- watching TV for long periods, particularly in the evening;
- eating, drinking or reading in bed.

Watching TV for long periods, both in the daytime and in the evening, is a habit that not only causes stiffness, but also interferes with sleep. This is because TV provokes numerous emotional responses in rapid succession, quickening the heart rate and releasing chemicals (such as adrenaline) for no useful purpose. When these chemicals are produced naturally, we deal with the situation and our blood flow is returned to normal. However, when chemicals are induced second-hand – such as occurs when watching TV – they remain in the bloodstream. This causes tension to linger, and ultimately gives rise to more stiffness and even muscle pain.

Wakefulness due to pain

Most people with arthritis find that once they are lying down and the stress has been taken off their joints, the pain slowly eases. This is not always the case, though, particularly when your hips and/or knees are affected and you are lying on your side. The only answer here may be for you to sleep all night on your back – at least until your self-help measures begin to alleviate the pain.

For the last 15 years I have had no choice but to lie on my back and I still don't always find this easy. If I roll on to my side accidentally, the pain in the soft tissues around the hips (from my fibromyalgia) wakes me and I need to turn on to my back once more. I must admit, though, that most of the time I manage to sleep quite well on my back – most things can be got used to, given time. If I am experiencing a period when getting off to sleep in this way is difficult, I take a warm bath before bedtime and this helps to relax me. I can then usually get off to sleep on my side without pain, turning on to my back some time later when the pain returns – but when I am sleepy enough to fall asleep again straight away.

Sleep medication

Any sleep problems associated with arthritis can be improved by taking a tricyclic antidepressant medication such as **imipramine, amitriptyline, doxepin, trazodone** or **lofepramine**. Tricyclic antidepressants are available from your doctor on prescription and work by increasing the concentration of chemicals that are known to promote sleep, reduce pain levels and ease muscle tension – you don't need to be depressed to gain benefits from them. To prevent the feeling of a 'thick head' the next morning, tricyclics are best taken in the evening rather than immediately before bedtime. The possible side effects include 'foggy brain', weight gain, constipation, dizziness, nausea, sweating, dry mouth, and short-term memory problems.

Over-the-counter sleep medications can increase the duration of sleep, but will not lengthen 'deep sleep' – the stage of sleep essential for tissue repair and regeneration. Tricyclic antidepressants (see above) can, however, encourage deep sleep. If you have been prescribed this kind of medication but it is no longer effective, the dosage may require adjusting or you may need to try another type.

Vitamin D3

If you have insomnia, it is possible to take a simple laboratory test to find out whether you are deficient in vitamin D3 – a hormone that is integral to the sleep process. It is best taken in liquid form and placed by a dropper on to your tongue before going to bed – 4,000 iu, taken in two 2,000 iu drops, seems to work best. If you are interested in trying this option, speak to your doctor.

5-HTP (hydroxy-tryptophan)

When vitamin D3 is taken in combination with a chemical called 5-HTP – which raises levels of a sleep-inducing chemical in the body called serotonin – sleep patterns can revert to normal within a few days. It is recommended that 100 mg to 200 mg of 5-HTP is taken daily with vitamin D3 until lab tests show that you are no longer deficient in the vitamin.

If you have depression as well as sleeplessness, you can take 100 mg dosages of 5-HTP three or four times daily without the need for lab tests beforehand. Depression often responds well to a return to the normal sleep rhythm, adrenal gland support (which 5-HTP offers), and vitamin and mineral therapy, as discussed in Chapter 5.

4

Help for your emotions

Arthritis can affect every area of your life. After diagnosis, it is common to be beset by fears for the future and anxieties about your effectiveness as a 'functioning' human being. How the people you care about will cope can also be a worry – after all, you want them to understand what's happening to you, but you don't wish to become a burden. Given time, education and self-awareness training, however, it is possible to adapt to the illness, and find ways of coping with the pain and stress. You can learn to focus on the present and recapture feelings of achievement by acquiring new interests and maybe, if you have a job, look for a less stressful post. The passing of time also allows others to see that you are trying your very best, and that you'll remain the same person inside.

Prolonged illness

Many people fail to appreciate that prolonged illness creates problems within the mind as well as within the body. Feelings of vulnerability, guilt, uselessness, fear and being out of control can taint our dealings with others, and be incredibly difficult to shake off.

'I feel so vulnerable'

Vulnerability is a natural human condition. We all need people to love us; we all crave the affirmation of others. To a large extent we are all dependent upon others too, measuring their responses in order to reassure ourselves that we are worthwhile human beings, and that we are indeed lovable. When we have a prolonged illness, as well as feeling unattractive we believe we have little to offer the people around us and so we fear we are no longer worthy of their love.

Feelings of vulnerability will always be present in so-called chronic illness, but we can defeat the worst of them by looking less to other people for affirmation. We all have inner strengths and particular talents, many of which we may be unaware of. Yet if we waited for others to point them out to us, we would likely be waiting for ever!

Your particular forte may be in planning and organizing, or problem solving, or handling finances (this doesn't necessarily have to be outside of the family either). You may be an authority on steam engines, an inspired cook, a good listener, a talented artist, an excellent singer, a diligent student, a competent driver, etc. Please do not underestimate yourself!

'I feel so guilty'

Feelings of guilt are common in prolonged illnesses. It is natural to want to lay the blame for becoming ill at someone's door, and many of us imagine we ourselves must have done something wrong to deserve such 'retribution'. But blaming either ourselves or others is pointless. Life is a lottery. Some of us inherit wealth, some don't; some inherit great intelligence, some don't; some fall ill and some remain healthy – that's just the way it is.

You may, after learning that improvement lies mainly in your own hands, feel guilty about making no real progress. However, assuming you have tried to help yourself, there is probably a sound reason for your lack of success. For example, you may have been unable to find enough information on exactly how to help yourself; you may be held back by additional health problems; or you may not have allowed sufficient time for any improvements to show.

Pain flare-ups are a perpetual threat in arthritis. When a flare-up has been caused by a chosen activity, you may well feel guilty. You may find viewing a flare-up as a 'painful' learning experience of some consolation – that is, you attempted to kneel down to polish the floor, but afterwards you were rigid with pain. Although it was a hard lesson, you learned that kneeling to polish the floor is bad for you.

Guilt also arises for those who feel they've become a burden on their families. For instance, they feel bad if they have caused their partner's workload to increase, if that person's free time has become limited, and if they seldom go out as a couple any more. When people with arthritis need a carer for much of the time, it is important that they realize that the carer (when it is a friend or family) needs time to himself or herself, to retain certain interests and have some 'time off'. The knowledge that your carer is enjoying life regardless of your less than perfect health and limitations – which, of course, he or she has a perfect right to do – should help you to feel less guilty.

'I feel so afraid'

Of course we are afraid when we have an illness for which there is, as yet, no absolute cure. Our fears tend to centre on the future and what will become of us. We are afraid of deteriorating further; afraid of becoming dependent upon others; afraid of the long-term effects of medication; afraid we will lose our friends . . . the list is endless.

It is not always easy to be cheerful and bright when you have a cold, never mind a painful condition to which you can see no end. At least you know that the cold will soon pass, and you can tell yourself that your spirits will then be restored. Those with arthritis do not have that comfort.

In most cases of arthritis, the fear of the unknown abates with time, however. You learn that you can still take pleasure from family life; you can still enjoy social occasions; you can still be of use to others; and you can take up new interests and hobbies. And in realizing that the majority of your fears are unfounded, you can get on with integrating your arthritis into 'who you are', and then concentrate on enjoying your life.

'I feel so useless'

Arthritis can be, without doubt, a limiting condition. Tasks that were once accomplished with ease have, after the onset of the arthritis, either to be performed with caution, or dropped altogether. More often than not, many jobs around the house have to be allocated to other family members – or to a paid cleaner if you can afford one. Onlookers may quip, 'Lucky you – having someone else do all that hard work!' They don't realize you would give anything to be able to clean the house thoroughly each and every day.

It is the same with many of the activities you previously enjoyed, and not necessarily ones requiring much effort. Some people with arthritis are unable to tilt their heads to read or write (myself included – although I am able to 'touch type' for up to three hours, split into three one-hour sessions throughout the day). Knitting, sewing, sketching – even such a 'trivial' task as filling the kettle – can cause similar problems, and may have to be set aside for the present. But don't give up hope of ever again being able to do these things, especially the activities you once enjoyed. The heaviest and most demanding of tasks may be permanently out of your scope, but other pleasures (and tasks) can be achieved given time and patience, and by the employment of pain- and stress-management strategies (see the end of this chapter).

'I feel so out of control'

Having little control over your arthritis may feel frightening. However, attempts at regaining a sense of control by, for example, dishing out orders from your wheelchair, or by interfering in other people's lives, are not a good idea!

In time, those with prolonged illnesses generally evolve their own coping strategies – many of which they may be unaware of – and they learn how to master certain situations. They may even end up having more control over their lives than beforehand, which is not a bad thing! For example, we can learn to control the way we talk to and respond to others; we can train our minds to focus on the present instead of the future; we can discipline ourselves to take health-related disappointments in our stride, and we can control our viewpoints, developing a more positive, realistic approach to life.

Arthritis and other people

When people ask how you are, yet respond to your replies with boredom, disbelief or even sarcasm, you may have got into the habit of muttering, 'I'm not too bad, thanks' or 'A bit better today . . .'. Unfortunately, conveying the nature, severity and complexity of arthritis to someone who sees it as only a 'slight problem' is, without doubt, very hard work. But if you are not straightforward, open and succinct – and the stark truth is that many listeners get bored when others 'harp on' about their maladies – I'm afraid that certain people around you may never understand.

'How can I make people understand?'

Sarcastic and derisory remarks from others can chip away at your confidence. Such comments should not, therefore, pass unchallenged. Standing up for yourself is not easy, but doing so can have a releasing effect – unlike when you fake indifference, or clam up and walk away. In these instances, you may end up feeling hurt, offended and very resentful. Your most intense feeling, however, will likely be that of anger – at the other person, and at yourself, for allowing yourself to be hurt.

If your partner were to complain, 'I do all the housework while you do nothing', I suggest you respond: 'I'm trying as hard as I can – but when I have a flare-up, everything I do makes me worse. I know it seems unfair when you're stuck with all the housework. It might help you to know that seeing you so busy upsets me, too. I really do appreciate your efforts, though. Perhaps we should learn to put up with a bit of dust and clutter.' If the initial comment was made during a heated exchange, you could answer, 'That's a hurtful thing to say. I may be doing very little, but it's not my fault. I'd like to talk this through when we're calmer.'

When family members are consistently sceptical of your condition – no matter what words or manner you employ – you may feel so hurt that you consider cutting yourself off from them completely. If their condemnations of you border on the fanatical, then this is perhaps your only choice. Otherwise, you would be best advised to keep steadily hammering away at your case, remembering to bring all unfair comments to their attention.

It may help you to know that when people close to you refuse to hear your assertions of ill health, it is often because they can't face the fact that a person that they love dearly is suffering. The only way they can deal with the illness is to refuse to believe in it. In effect, they cope by *not* coping. But that is their problem, not yours. Don't ever give up on them, though, for almost everything changes with time.

Sadly, it's the people outside of your immediate circle who can be the most cutting in their remarks. Again, they have no right to hurt you, nor should they get away with it. Your best weapons here are words that make them think. For example, a person who asks mockingly, 'Are we any better today?' could be met with, 'Is there something on your mind? If so, just say it. If you really are concerned about my health, thank you. The truth is my knee is hurting terribly, and I don't know how I'll manage to get home.'

Those with arthritis frequently face remarks such as, 'I noticed you went shopping last Saturday. I thought you weren't able to walk far?' or 'I saw you in the pub on Sunday. Your arthritis can't be that bad!' In such situations, replies could go along the lines of, 'Yes, I did manage to get out last weekend. I have good days and bad. But even though I was feeling better, the effort brought the inflammation back and I had to rest all week afterwards.'

'Why have I lost so many friends?'

As you may already have discovered, having a prolonged condition leaves you in little doubt as to who your real friends are. The 'friends' who are offended when you break an appointment, the 'friends' who are unconvinced when you explain that, yes, you were able to have a night out with them last week, but you are not up to going out tonight, and, worst still, the 'friends' who complain that you have again let them down are really not worth your precious energy. Any negative input into your life is detrimental to your confidence as well as to your stress levels and sense of wellbeing.

It's natural to feel guilty when you think you've let someone down. You shouldn't, though, let that spur you into attempting an activity you know will be to your detriment – for example, turning up at the next social event despite stiffness and pain, and despite knowing that doing so is likely to make you worse.

Placing yourself at risk in this way is really not worth temporarily assuaging your guilt. Before going ahead with any activity, your main considerations should be your own physical and emotional health. In other words, you should only embark on something when doing so is for your own good and not someone else's.

And what about the 'friends' who, after you have been unable to socialize as before, have gradually dropped out of your life? Can you honestly say they were true friends? Wouldn't a true friend make allowances for your arthritis? Wouldn't a true friend try to understand what you were going through?

Speaking to others

If you are speaking to someone who clearly cares about your health, it's important that your responses are clear and open. You may wish to describe how you feel emotionally, in which case you need to focus on how you actually do feel. It may be difficult to admit you feel guilty, frustrated, angry, useless, vulnerable, etc., even to yourself. Sharing your feelings with other people can be even harder, yet it is an important step towards halting the problems that those feelings can cause. In your need to be understood by others, however, you should be wary of making assumptions regarding how they feel about you.

It's the people we care deeply about whom we *most* want to understand how we are feeling. Speaking to someone in the following way, though, is sure to cause offence: 'I get upset when you think I'm exaggerating!' or 'I don't believe you really care about me, and that makes me feel so hopeless!' or 'I'm losing confidence because you treat me as if I'm not trying to help myself!' Such comments are likely to be seen as accusations, and they may even provoke a quarrel.

Speaking directly of the way you feel – without implying that the other person is contributing to any problems you have – will incline them to take your comments more seriously. It should encourage them to be more thoughtful, too.

It is best to take the following into account before attempting to speak openly of your feelings:

• Ensure you have interpreted the other person's behaviour correctly. For example, you may view your mother bringing you a basket of fruit and vegetables as a criticism of your diet – when in truth it is a goodwill gesture, just to show she cares! You have a perfect right to interpret the words or actions of others in whatever way you wish, but that interpretation is not necessarily reality. In fact, it is amazing how wrong we often are in our perceptions of what others think and feel.

- Make sure you are specific in recalling another person's behaviour. For example, 'You never understand how exhausted I get' is far more inflammatory than 'You didn't seem to understand yesterday, when I told you how exhausted I was'.
- Ensure that what you are about to say is what you really mean. For example, statements such as, 'Everyone thinks you're insensitive' and 'We all think you've got an attitude problem' are, besides being inflammatory, very unfair. We have no way of knowing that 'everyone' is of the same opinion. The use of the depersonalized 'everyone', 'we' or 'us' – often said in the hope of deflecting the listener's anger – can cause more hurt and anger than if the criticism was personal.

It's easy to see how others can misunderstand or take offence when we fail to communicate effectively. Changing the habits of a lifetime is not easy, though, for it means analysing our thoughts before rearranging them into speech. But we are rewarded for our efforts when people start to listen and when they cease to be annoyed as we carefully explain an area they don't fully understand.

Dealing with co-workers

If you are managing to work and cope with arthritis at the same time, well done! Allowances or exceptions being made in the workplace for those with prolonged ill health generally have to be fought for. And even if you have an understanding boss, colleagues are often less tolerant.

If your employers are not yet making allowances for your arthritis, simply be honest with them and don't be tempted to cover up any health-related shortcomings. Those who do and are found out are rarely shown leniency. Indeed, unless you are unable to communicate the nature of your illness and how it affects your performance, you are liable to be condemned as slow and inefficient – especially by your co-workers who may be convinced you are not pulling your weight.

It's a fact that, given sufficient information about your condition, employers can be more sympathetic than certain fellow employees. Your exclusion from certain duties may even prompt others to make snide remarks, usually prompted by jealousy, resentment, distrust, or simply because you are an easy target when they are having a bad day. Snide remarks, however, are cruel and unjust and should not be tolerated.

The thought of objecting to an unfair accusation, particularly when you are at a low ebb, may seem daunting – but as well as being the only means of getting through to some people, it also helps you to maintain self-esteem. For example, a co-worker may remark, 'You're looking fine. Are you sure you're not using your arthritis to get out of doing all the lifting?' Whether the tone is light or not, the content is unwarranted. Failing to respond – maybe because you are too angry or too hurt – only serves to confirm their opinion, I'm afraid. Therefore, your answer should be a firm, 'I resent that. I'm glad you think I look OK – but I would certainly never use my arthritis as an excuse.' The other person will usually apologize at this point, and may even confess, 'I suppose I just don't understand properly what's wrong with you.' Here is your chance to explain further about your condition.

When the people around you appear to be in a receptive frame of mind, try to grasp the opportunity to explain your arthritis. Your symptoms may best be understood when you equate them to something within the listener's experience. For instance, to someone who enjoys climbing, you could say, 'The stiffness makes me feel like I climbed Everest yesterday', or, to someone who has experienced sports injuries, 'The pain in my shoulder is like a torn ligament'. Descriptive analogies can be effective, too (so long as you don't go over the top): 'The pain is like having a nagging toothache, but in my hip' or 'When I walk, it feels as if my joints are grinding together at the knee' makes the listener really think.

Dealing with negative thinking

When people frequently voice the same negative thoughts, it usually means they are afraid of the very thing about which they are being negative. The mother who decries weakness in most cases does it because she secretly fears she is weak. The father who denounces incompetence in most cases has deep-seated doubts about his own competence. When their offspring copy these attitudes into adulthood, condemning weakness and incompetence as well as displaying other negative viewpoints, this too stems from inherent beliefs that they are lacking in certain ways.

Our mindsets – that is, either trust or distrust, enthusiasm or depression, self-assurance or timidity, anxiety or serenity, etc. – usually arise from childhood conditioning. Consequently, our automatic thoughts are determined by whatever mindsets have been built into our character, controlling our behaviour in any given situation. For example, when planning a birthday party, a person with a depressive mindset would dread the 'big day', worrying that few guests would even turn up. A person with an enthusiastic mindset, on the other hand, would eagerly await the party, sure of its success. A person with a trustful mindset would regard the comment 'That sweater's a bit small for you, love' as a caring remark and happily change into something that fitted better. A person with a distrustful mindset, on the other hand, would take it as a criticism of his or her weight, of the sweater, of his or her choice of attire, or of all these put together!

Irrational feelings

Negative mindsets invariably produce irrational feelings about ourselves, and these feelings tend to become 'self-fulfilling prophecies'. For example, 'I will never be any good with money' stops us trying to be effective with money. 'I will never make anyone happy' stops us trying to make anyone happy, and, concerning ill health, 'I am no fun to have around any more' makes us stop trying to retain good humour when we're with others. These irrational feelings are actually *untruths* that determine behaviour.

But irrational feelings can be turned around, and a more positive approach can be learned. First, though, it's important to acknowledge irrational thoughts and feelings for what they are, and for the behaviour they induce. Forthcoming family celebrations commonly provoke feelings of anxiety in people with prolonged illnesses. However, actually writing down your negative thoughts and feelings and really analysing them can make the fact that they are irrational crystal clear. It makes you more aware.

An example of possible irrational thoughts and feelings prior to a family party is given in Table 1.

The examples in Table 1 illustrate just how irrational prolonged ill health can, at times, make someone. Yet without analysis, the potential repercussions can be staggering. In this situation, you may end up talking yourself into staying at home, experiencing mixed self-pity, guilt, and even self-loathing. Your decision could even cause an argument with your partner.

If you are no worse than usual, then, realistically, staying at home is hardly the answer. Indeed, no matter how dire your 'normal' condition, you must, for the sake of your sanity, have a life; you need to be with others occasionally and therefore make an extra effort every now and again. Given sufficient forward planning, certain events really can be managed effectively, for whether your symptoms are severe or not, backing out of events and activities you may have enjoyed can leave you feeling angry at yourself, furious with your illness, and resentful that everyone else is in good health!

I was taught by a pain psychologist to record my thoughts and feelings prior to a difficult event, and doing so always helps me. Assuming, then, that you are no worse than usual, try to write down your expectations about what will happen at the party (in the format given in Table 1). Now look objectively at what you have written. Are your thoughts and feelings reasonable? Surely you would feel like a wet-blanket if you sat with a face as long

Table 1 Possible irrational thoughts and feelings prior to a family party

Situation	Irrational thoughts	Irrational feelings
Family party.	I will be a real wet blanket. No one will want to talk to me. I will put a dampener on the whole event.	I will then feel sad and alienated. I will hate myself for being such a misery.

as a fiddle and made no effort to talk to anyone! And could you really be so impolite that you would avoid conversing? Are your relatives really so antisocial they would disregard you? When we challenge negative feelings thus, the reality of the situation soon becomes apparent. People do make an effort to be friendly at family gatherings. Your fellow guests are people you know well. Common ground can always be found, should you wish to look for it.

So, you have re-evaluated and subsequently vanquished one set of negative thoughts – but perhaps only to find it replaced by another? You have decided to attend the party, but now you are worrying about coping with pain in company. Will the pain totally consume you? Will you burst into tears? Will everyone think you pathetic?

Although it is normal to worry about coping with pain when out of your usual environment, your worries may, due to your fears, be somewhat distorted. Writing them down helps you see them in a more detached light.

In Table 2, I have incorporated a column listing possible solutions.

Table 2 Possible solutions to irrational thoughts and feelings

Situation	Irrational thoughts	Irrational feelings	Solution
'I will be in a lot of pain at the party.'	'I will be unable to cope with the pain. I will feel as if I could cry. I will get angry and accuse everyone of not caring.'	'People will think me weak and stupid. They will hate me for spoiling the occasion. I will then feel angry with myself.'	'I will take painkillers before leaving and take more with me for later. I'll ask to lie down if I start to feel bad.'

In Table 2, irrational feelings are seen for what they are, and possible solutions are considered. Other solutions may include choosing the most supportive chair, asking for an ice pack or bag of frozen peas to place over a painful area, or explaining in advance that you may have to leave early. After all, looking for realistic ways in which to ease a difficult situation is far more helpful than immersing yourself in worries that will probably get you nowhere. More importantly, it can help you to cope with some degree of pain.

You may then find yourself assailed by further worries. You have planned to ask if you may lie down for half an hour, but when the time comes, you feel too anxious to do so. Surely your hosts will think you feeble and demanding? Surely everyone will stare and whisper behind your back? This again is irrational thinking and, since obviously it won't always be convenient for you to write down your feelings, you should mentally consider what you need to do. In this instance, all you can do, unless you want to risk incurring thoughts of self-loathing and self-pity – on top of a certain increase in pain – is pluck up your nerve and ask.

From my own personal experience, I can honestly say that most people are only too willing to assist when asked directly. Often they haven't been sure what help to offer, but when you ask for help, it takes the pressure off them. They will likely then want to know whether the bedroom is warm enough, the bed firm enough, the pillows soft enough . . . If they do scowl and make a comment to the effect that you are making a fuss – and in all my years of asking others for help regarding my own maladies, I have never come across anyone who has – it says a lot more about his or her nature than anything about yours!

Advice for parents of children with arthritis

When your child has juvenile RA (JRA) – or any other form of arthritis – the whole family is affected. Parents are anxious, the child is likely to be miserable, angry or simply confused, and siblings may swing between anxiety and jealousy – the anxiety transferring from their parents, the jealousy because their brother or sister receives more attention than they themselves do. Arthritis can also make classwork difficult. It can compromise a young person's participation in school games and social activities, too.

To help the child cope emotionally and get the most out of life physically, it is recommended that family members do the following:

- Treat the child as normally as possible.
- As some children think their arthritis is a punishment for something they did wrong, explain that becoming ill is nobody's fault.
- Ensure that the child receives good medical care. Arthritis can affect children very differently, so it is not a case of 'one medication fitting all'. There are actually several available medications and if your child fails to respond well to one or experiences side effects, you should discuss other options with the doctor. When symptoms are controlled, the child can be more active.
- Encourage appropriate social development. Some children may only be able to partake in social activities when they are free of symptoms – however, it is important that they interact with other children during flare-ups as well, if at all possible. This could involve inviting one or two children to your house so they can all play computer or board games together.
- When the child is well enough, ensure that he or she takes exercise in the form of school games, playing outside with friends, and partaking in team sports. This helps to keep the joints strong and supple and encourages appropriate social development. Swimming is a particularly good activity for people with arthritis as it works many muscles and joints without stressing them too much.
- Ensure that the child is referred by a doctor to attend regular physiotherapy sessions. Encourage him or her to perform the recommended daily exercise programme at home too – the physiotherapist will teach this. If the child is in too much pain to carry out the programme, ensure that he or she doesn't try to make up for lost time later. The programme should be recommenced very carefully, performing fewer repetitions than before and slowly building up to where they had been.
- Ensure that the child's teacher is educated about juvenile arthritis, and that he or she makes sure all the children in the class are well informed – perhaps by sending the children home with an informative letter. If the teacher is not willing to do this, try to educate other parents so they will inform

their children – that is, consider writing brief letters to the parents.

- Although most children with arthritis progress normally through school, make sure that the teacher sends assignments home, especially when the child is absent for long periods.
- If there is a support group for children with juvenile arthritis in your area, consider joining it. This gives affected children the opportunity to share experiences with others 'in the same boat'. Coping techniques can also be passed on, helping both the child and his or her family to manage the situation.

5

Environmental toxins

Although it is generally accepted that arthritis has a hereditary component – in other words, it is often passed down through the family – some experts believe the condition is also connected with exposure to chemical stressors in the environment. These are often referred to as 'allergens'.

Indoor air contaminants (or allergens) include building materials, paints, varnish, glues, deodorizers, plastics, carpeting, insecticides, disinfectants, sulphites, chlorine, formaldehyde, mould, detergents, dyes, and gas leakage from stoves and heaters. Synthetic drugs – that is, those derived from petroleum – are a common source of sensitivity too. Personal care products such as deodorants, skin lotions, nail polish, cosmetics, perfumes, shower gels, shampoo and conditioners etc. can also provoke adverse reactions in sensitive individuals. Biologically friendly products are now available at certain High Street chemists, and from some suppliers of nutritional supplements.

As we saw on page 12, it was Dr Theron Randolph who first developed the theory that chemical stressors in the environment can cause illness in sensitive people. He explained to his arthritis patients that non-organic foods containing chemical additives could create inflammation, and is said to have guided them in removing their specific 'problem foods' from their diets (see page 79 for information on how to do this yourself). He claims to have witnessed huge improvements in many people as a result. Dr Randolph later included environmental pollutants such as chemical pesticides and cleaning fluids in his warnings, advising his patients that they would improve further if they also removed these from their everyday lives. There are testaments from some of his patients (not all) to suggest that their improvement was substantial – however, the experiment was not classed as a proper scientifically controlled study.

More recently, allergy specialist Dr John Mansfield claimed impressive results after a large number of his arthritis patients trialled what he refers to as 'ecological treatment'. This was basically the same regime as advocated by Dr Randolph, involving a toxin-free diet – that is, organic foods with no chemical additives – and removing as many everyday pollutants as possible.

Unfortunately, neither of the above experiments was viewed with the gravitas of properly controlled scientific studies. It would actually be incredibly difficult, if not impossible, to carry out a long-term scientific experiment in which intake and environment are carefully controlled, for the participants would each require monitoring 24 hours a day. It is not yet clear whether there can ever be any recognized study results to prove the merits of a toxin-free regime. Until such recognized studies take place – if they ever do – I believe that experts must make their own judgements from the existing experiments, and hope that more are carried out in the near future.

Exposure to chemical stressors

Some individuals appear to be more susceptible than others to chemical stressors (allergens) – especially those with illnesses such as arthritis and those with other types of immune system dysfunction.

Dr William Meggs from North Carolina in the USA is currently researching chemical sensitivities, and indoor exposure to various substances. His carefully observed beliefs about the stages of chemically induced illness are outlined below:

- Stage 0 – **tolerance**: this is the state of being able to cope with your chemical environment.
- Stage 1 – **sensitization**: this is the state of being irritated by chemical exposure. It is common for the person to say they are 'allergic' to certain substances which produce symptoms such as headache, fatigue, nausea, muscle pain, joint pain, hives and so on.
- Stage 2 – **inflammation**: this stage occurs when chemical exposure leads to tissue inflammation conditions such as arthritis, vasculitis, colitis, myositis, rhinitis, some types of dermatitis and so on. At this stage, unless tissue damage

has already occurred, the inflammation can be reversed by removal of the offending agent. Stage 2 symptoms can be controlled by some medications, unless the person is sensitive to them. Medications are not a cure for chemical sensitivity, however. Indeed, there is always the risk of Stage 2 symptoms recurring and even progressing to Stage 3 if the offending chemical substance is not removed.

• Stage 3 – **tissue and organ deterioration**: in this stage, the constant onslaught of chemical stressors has given rise to chronic inflammation and damage to some tissues – that is, perhaps in the nerves, kidneys, liver, lungs and autoimmune system (see below for more detail). Sadly, this stage is irreversible and correct function of the organ is lost. Please note that people can reach Stage 3 without ever linking their problems to chemical sensitivities. However, even if you think you are in Stage 3 as defined by Dr Meggs, it is still not too late to evaluate your environment for possible contributing factors. It's important that you also make certain lifestyle changes to prevent further deterioration.

Organophosphates

Organophosphates (known as OPs), which are now widely used in farming practices throughout the Western world, give rise to one of the most common chemical sensitivities. OPs are highly toxic chemicals used regularly for pest control in crop production and animal husbandry. They are also present in home pesticides such as fly sprays etc. OPs were originally developed to attack the central nervous system in order to kill during warfare. They can adversely affect every bodily system and are believed to be implicated in the onset of arthritis. Note that OPs are never used in organic farming, however.

Typical symptoms of OP poisoning include mental and physical fatigue, poor muscle stamina, muscle pain, drug intolerance, irritable bowel syndrome, sweating, low body temperature, numb areas, muscle twitching, clumsiness, mood swings, irritability, short-term memory problems and poor concentration. It's possible to rid your body of OPs by avoiding exposure to them, by following an organic diet, and by taking antioxidant supplements. Vitamins A, C and E, vitamin B12, magnesium and selenium are particularly effective.

Heavy metals

In addition to chemicals, our bodies are constantly absorbing small quantities of heavy metals every day. The worst culprits are as follows:

Aluminium

Because high levels of aluminium cause damage to the central nervous system, it is believed to be implicated in the onset of many illnesses. Sources of aluminium poisoning may be aluminium cookware, foil, containers and underarm deodorants. This metal can also be found in coffee, bleached white flour and some antacid medications. Interestingly, experts now believe that magnesium and calcium deficiencies increase the toxic effects of ingested aluminium.

Mercury

Individuals with amalgam tooth fillings are ingesting minute amounts of mercury vapour every day, which can gradually weaken their immune systems. Synthetic white fillings are a safe alternative. Mercury fillings must be removed with great care.

Lead

Ingested lead is known to cause neurological and psychological disturbance. Some old houses still have lead piping, others have copper piping fused together with lead-based solder. The use of a water-filter device is highly recommended in cases like this – although, obviously, replacing the old piping with modern copper or synthetic piping is far safer.

Cadmium

High carbohydrate consumption is now thought to be linked with raised cadmium levels in the body. Cigarette-smoking is another cause of cadmium build-up, cadmium being mainly absorbed through the lungs. This metal is known to be damaging to the kidneys and lungs. It can, however, be gradually removed by a detoxification diet, followed by good nutrition.

A food elimination programme

Discovering whether you are sensitive to a particular food can be difficult, and each of the blood and skin tests available can be found fault with by experts. The only certain way to prove the case is via a food elimination programme. However, to eliminate one food at a time, then to have to wait in order to assess your body's response, would take many months. For this reason, attending an allergy clinic is advisable. The test results will at least point you in the right direction.

Foods that most often cause sensitivity reactions include pork, beef, chicken, cow's milk products, wheat, egg, alcohol, corn, nuts, tomato, chocolate, citrus fruits and mushrooms. Pork is actually closely linked with arthritis and is, for many, a major cause of inflammatory flare-ups. In fact, as red meats are often involved in triggering arthritic pain, some experts recommend a mainly vegetarian diet with small amounts of poultry and oily fish.

If you have an idea which foods are causing you problems, there is no reason for you not to test out your instincts, removing them from your diet for a period of one month. This can save you a great deal of money and time. Recent studies on people with RA indicated that 30–40 per cent are likely to benefit from excluding certain suspect foods from their diet.

Food sensitivity versus food allergy

Bear in mind that many people are sensitive to the foods they most often consume, the result perhaps being persistent headaches or stomach upsets. It's even possible to have a true addiction to one or more foods, meaning that removing it can make you feel quite ill for a few days. Of course, returning to the old ways will immediately perk you up, just as smoking a cigarette again will immediately boost someone who is trying to quit. Note, though, that true food allergies create a range of severe symptoms that can even be life-threatening. It is essential, therefore, that you track down the allergen by looking at what you ate directly before the allergic reaction. This foodstuff must then be eliminated from your diet.

If you believe you are allergic rather than just sensitive to some foods – a true allergy is far more serious than a sensitivity – it is probably best that instead of DIY testing, you speak to your doctor about the possibility of testing at an allergy clinic. Here, should anaphalactic shock occur – this is when the respiratory tract becomes inflamed and breathing erratic – immediate expert treatment is to hand. Anaphalactic shock is not a common allergic reaction, but it does happen on occasion.

During the elimination process

During a food elimination programme, it is important to eat only organically produced foods. This is because some people react badly to the pesticides and other chemicals used in non-organic farming. The chlorine in tap water can cause problems too, which makes it best to drink only spring water during the month-long protocol. It is even possible to be sensitive to plastic, hence you should avoid plastic bottles and purchase only glass ones. An alternative is to boil tap water for 20 minutes – it is then safe to drink it.

Assuming your suspicions are correct regarding your problem foods, there is often an initial withdrawal reaction in the form of fatigue, headaches, twitching and irritability – which can persist for up to 15 days. Drinking at least five pints of water daily helps to reduce withdrawal symptoms; it also aids detoxification and helps to flush any residual toxins through the digestive tract.

A hypersensitive stage can then follow this period. Indeed, if you unwittingly eat an irritant food that you are attempting to eliminate, the ensuing reaction can be severe, particularly when true allergy is the problem. When dining out, it is recommended that you ask the chef, not the waiter, if you are unsure about the ingredients.

On a brighter note, a pleasing symptom of withdrawal can be weight loss. The reason for this – assuming you are not starving yourself, which would be completely wrong and unnecessary – is that many people with food sensitivities have an unrecognized excess of fluid distributed throughout their bodies in the form of swelling (inflammation). When they begin to remove all traces of the offending foods from their bodies, the excess fluid quickly drains away.

If you think you may be short of important vitamins and minerals during the month-long elimination process, you may be able to replace them by eating more cereal, vegetables, liver and fish (assuming these are not the foods you think you could be allergic to). You can also take vitamins from the B group (which are known to be 'allergy'-friendly). All the fruit you eat should first be thoroughly washed, dried, peeled and eaten immediately.

Elimination and re-introduction strategy

By the end of the month many of you will feel better than you have for a long time. This feeling of wellbeing can be so great that you won't want to bother to re-introduce the excluded foods.

But for those who do wish to re-introduce these foods, a procedure is suggested in Table 3.

Table 3 Re-introducing excluded foods

Day 1	In the morning, re-introduce a small amount of a food or drink previously eliminated (not a full-sized portion). Do the same later in the day. Record any symptoms.
Day 2	If you don't experience symptoms, repeat the exercise. Once again, record any symptoms you do have. If you get through the second day, this is really good news! Well done!

Now wait for two more days before you can safely re-introduce this food into your diet on a fairly regular basis.
Repeat the above four-day re-introduction procedure with each food eliminated.

Any side effects should have occurred within four days. You may feel disappointed, though, if your problem is not intolerance but turns out to be true allergy. True allergies cause an *immediate* reaction – that is, the immune system responds as if it is being invaded, setting up antibodies to the offending food(s). Obviously you will need to avoid this food on a permanent basis.

If you do experience symptoms – say, for example, you develop a headache after re-introducing cheese – it would be better to avoid eating cheese for at least six months before attempting to re-introduce it. However, some foods will always cause an adverse reaction, so it would be wise to withdraw them from your diet altogether.

As bread, cakes, etc. contain a mixture of ingredients, using the elimination and re-introduction strategy wouldn't show which ingredient was causing you a problem. To assess whether you are sensitive to wheat in particular, it is best, therefore, to cut out cereal products and instead eat crackers containing only wheat and salt. If you still experience a reaction, you will know wheat is the culprit and you will need to avoid it for at least the next six months.

In the meantime, continue to eat sensibly. Try not to indulge too much in the foods that previously caused problems. And remember, if in doubt, leave it out!

Lack of vitamin and mineral absorption

Slow food absorption may be the underlying problem in people with multiple food sensitivities. This usually means that essential vitamins and minerals are slow to be absorbed too – and, consequently, this will result in deficiencies. This particularly applies to the water-soluble B group, and also vitamin C.

If you suspect that slow absorption applies to you, speak to your doctor. You may need to take supplements on a long-term basis, and they may be available on prescription. If not, look for good-quality supplements, such as those from the manufacturers recommended in the Useful addresses section at the back of this book.

Multiple food sensitivities

If you have multiple food sensitivities and need to avoid eating a wide range of foods, you are likely to be deficient in important minerals such as magnesium, calcium, potassium, zinc and iron. To counter the deficiencies, it is advisable that you visit your doctor – you may be offered multi-vitamin and multi-mineral supplements on prescription.

The way we were

Where diet is concerned, we now eat a wide variety of processed foods – that is, foods grown with the use of toxic chemicals and with added artificial preservatives, flavourings, colourings, etc. Yet our bodies, physiologically speaking, have barely changed since cave man times. They were certainly not built to cope with all the toxins we put into them.

Cave man's digestive system was fairly simple, as were the foods they were eating at the time. The foods were not sprayed with chemicals or injected with preservatives, they were eaten fresh and in season – and fresh, uncontaminated fruit and vegetables are highly nutritious. They are also rich in **enzymes**, the substances that aid digestion. For the most part, the food was uncooked, too, which is the best way to eat it. Cooking at a temperature above 41°C (107°F) destroys live digestive enzymes, which help to break down the food. Refrigeration has a similarly destructive effect.

Foodstuffs today

So-called 'modern man' has developed the following habits:

• We eat food grown on artificially fertilized land and sprayed several times with chemical pesticides. This destroys essential soil microbes that would otherwise help plants to absorb the nutrient-rich minerals essential to good health.
• Plant foods are then artificially ripened, stored and processed.
• We eat foods out of season, because they are readily available.
• We eat the tasty parts of the food only, disposing of the rest. For example, wheat husks are removed before the remaining cereal is processed into white flour. When food is left 'whole', it aids the removal of waste materials from the bowel. Thus 'wholefoods' are vital to good digestive and bowel health.

Food recommendations for those with arthritis

To help your body start healing itself, it requires a wide variety of foods and food combinations. This helps to ensure you are ingesting a wide range of essential vitamins, minerals and fatty acids. To eat the same foods repeatedly means missing out on many important building blocks of life, for certain foods build and regenerate only certain parts of the body.

Because the majority of our foodstuffs are grown in a chemical environment, they are low in nutrients and high in toxicity. It is advisable, therefore, to purchase organically grown produce, and to look for foods without added artificial chemicals (colourings, flavourings, preservatives, etc.).

Here are some guidelines for eating an improved diet:

- Avoid missing meals. When we allow ourselves to become very hungry, then sugary, high-fat foods become more tempting.
- Minimize your sugar intake. Use raw honey, date sugar, molasses, barley malt etc. in place of table sugar and artificial sweeteners such as aspartame and saccharin.
- Junk food and fast foods are loaded with harmful additives. Avoid them if at all possible.
- Look out for chemical additives on food labels. Flavourings, colourings and preservatives are often presented as 'E' numbers.
- Avoid refined and processed foods. Those that come in tins, jars and packets almost certainly contain additives (except for most foods purchased in healthfood shops). Fresh foodstuffs, on the other hand, are usually additive-free.
- Try to drink up to eight glasses of water a day, inclusive of fruit and/or vegetable juices and herbal teas. Distilled or filtered water is highly recommended.
- Ensure you are not consuming large quantities of salt, both in cooking and at the table. Remember that salt is commonly used as a preservative and added to most processed, pre-packaged foods. Rock salt and sea salt are healthier alternatives, but should still be used sparingly.
- Only take medication when you really need to. This will reduce the number of unnecessary toxins entering your body.
- Take the recommended vitamin and mineral supplements. Because people with arthritis have many nutritional deficiencies, supplements – tablet-form concentrates of a particular vitamin, mineral, etc. – are essential.
- Take antioxidant supplements to protect the cells and boost energy release.

How to locate problem chemicals in your environment

It can be difficult to pinpoint which environmental chemicals are causing you problems, if any. The fact some symptoms 'go underground' – that is, not showing up in a direct result of exposure to a particular substance – can make it even more difficult to link cause and effect. The best way of uncovering any offending agents is to follow an elimination programme similar to that used to reveal problem foods (see pages 79–82). You can do this by avoiding known problem chemicals, one by one, until you find one that makes you unwell in some way. Obviously, if at all possible, you should then remove this chemical from your immediate environment.

Another means of locating problem chemicals is by taking a break – usually for several weeks – by staying elsewhere for that period. Moving house is also a common way to escape an allergen. However, it still may not be easy to work out what was causing the problem.

The following are stories of four fortunate people who were able to pinpoint their particular 'nemeses' (though I need to reiterate here that not all arthritis is caused or exacerbated by environmental chemicals).

Tom

Having had arthritis in his knees for two years, 71-year-old Tom, an ex-joiner, decided to check his home for any chemicals that might be worsening his condition. First he threw away his much-used fly-killer, but after waiting a month there was no change in his symptoms. Next went his personal care products such as shower gel, shampoo, deodorants and after-shave, and instead he purchased biologically friendly products from a High Street pharmacy. Again, though, he could see no obvious change in his symptoms. He had high hopes about disposing of the glues and so on he used for his joinery, stored in the workshop attached to the house – but although his knees felt a little better for using nails, screws and other joinery techniques instead of glue, the improvement was not enough for his liking.

At last his gaze fell on the old gas heater that was invariably lit when he was working on the small ornamental wheelbarrows which had become his hobby. He substituted the old heater for a small electric one and his pain virtually disappeared within weeks. After taking the old heater to the tip, he purchased a carbon-dioxide detector to prevent such an event recurring with other gas appliances.

Polly

Polly, who is 37, had had arthritis for four years, but she noticed she felt much better for a change of environment – that is, two months at her brother's farm in Northumberland. But since her symptoms still made a partial return every time she entered her brother's bathroom when it was steamy, she suspected that being away from the stresses of her usual life was not the entire answer. Noticing that the bathmat and shower curtain were quite mouldy, she bought her brother new ones and, to her delight, found she improved dramatically.

Once back home, Polly suddenly noticed that the outer wall of her master bedroom was quite mouldy and damp, and the wallpaper was hanging off in the corner. She noticed too that there was thick black mould around the wooden window frame. With her father's help, she removed all the traces of mould – and within a few months she was her old self again. Aware now that mould, damp and humidity were her triggering agents, Polly resolved to keep her life as free of them as possible in future – even taking short showers instead of indulging in her usual long soak in the bath. She also took this opportunity to clean up her life, both dietary-wise and in the products she bought for personal and home use. She never looked back.

Elaine

Elaine, 62, had been troubled by arthritis for over ten years, but her symptoms eased after she moved out of her daughter Jodie's house. Jodie was an artist who, among other things, made papier-mâché, constructions for parades and other community events. Elaine now realized there was something about her daughter's home that was exacerbating her symptoms, since every time she visited Jodie her symptoms reappeared with a vengeance. She strongly suspected that Jodie's art materials – glues, varnish, paints, dyes and cleaning fluids – were responsible, so Elaine used some of the money she had saved in sharing the rent over the years to fund the building of a studio in Jodie's garden (Jodie had worked in the dining room up to that point). Once the many fumes from her daughter's artwork were contained in the studio, Elaine's symptoms stayed reasonably mild with very few flare-ups. The flare-ups became even less, however, when Elaine changed to an organic, additive-free diet and removed all allergens from her own home.

Mike

After 54-year-old Mike had experienced joint pains for a year, his doctor diagnosed arthritis. Mike didn't give a second thought to the fact that the pain actually began shortly after he and his wife moved into a house that was newly carpeted. However, he did think it strange that the pain eased a lot after the carpets downstairs were removed and oak floors laid instead. His wife insisted that they had new wooden flooring upstairs as well to see if he improved further. As a result, Mike's continued improvement was quite dramatic, and he decided to throw himself into the chemical-elimination programme, changing to eating only organic, additive-free foods and avoiding fabric softeners, air fresheners, scented candles and such. Before too long, he found himself virtually pain-free and was happy to have made adjustments to his life for the sake of his health.

Moving to another area?

Of course, not all allergens are so easy to get away from. Car exhaust fumes, for example, are a menace in all urban areas and around all major roads in the UK. Moving to the countryside could resolve an adverse reaction to them, but this entails drastic upheaval for all the family and requires careful consideration. For instance, if you would still need to drive into town to do your shopping or go to work, then your exposure to car exhaust fumes might be almost as great as it was before.

However, if the allergen is contained to one area – for instance, if you live close to a factory that emits chemical irritants – you could move to a cleaner area. Note, though, that it is against the law for any premises to release high amounts of pollutant into the atmosphere. You may be able to tackle the matter head-on by complaining about this to the environmental health department and maybe by speaking to your neighbours and drawing up a petition.

Medication

Some people even have an adverse reaction to a prescription medication. The reaction can vary from a mild localized rash to nausea, vomiting or diarrhoea if you are sensitive to a chemical in the drug. If you have a true allergy to a chemical in the drug, though, serious, life-threatening effects on the body can occur.

True allergic reactions only take place in about 10 per cent of cases, whereas sensitivity reactions account for around 90 per cent of cases.

Drug reactions can be caused by:

- an interaction between the new drug and others you take;
- an inability of the body to completely break down the chemicals in the drug; people with liver and kidney damage may have this problem;
- taking an overdose of the drug (whether accidentally or otherwise).

You should always visit your doctor when you experience a reaction to a particular medication, explaining what happened as best you can. Try not to use the word 'allergy' unless you are certain that a true allergic reaction took place. Some reactions may simply be a usual 'side effect' which should diminish in a short time. Note that if you are in any doubt as to whether you experienced a side effect or a drug reaction, you should still see your doctor. That's what they are there for.

The medications most likely to cause reactions are as follows:

- painkillers (analgesics) such as **morphine**, **codeine** and non-steroidal anti-inflammatory drugs (NSAIDs). The latter include **ibuprofen, indomethacin** and **aspirin.**
- anti-seizure medications such as **carbamazepine** and **phenytoin.**

6

Nutrition for arthritis

Although there is a great deal of advice around about diet for arthritis, not one diet has yet been proven (in properly controlled scientific studies) to be of benefit. The reason for this could simply be that it is incredibly difficult to control what a group of individuals consume over a set period. Currently, the favoured means of assessing whether a diet is effective is to look at all the available evidence, as mentioned below.

Nutritionists are keen to point out that diets advocating the elimination of vital food groups may be harmful. Many arthritis diets are certainly contradictory, with one recommending one type of food and another advising against the same one. This makes for a confusing state of affairs all round, meaning few people know what to eat for the best.

The anti-inflammatory diet

In 2009, after becoming interested in the idea that diet can play a role in preventing inflammation, Professor Philip Calder and his team at the University of Southampton scrutinized all the evidence in favour of consuming an anti-inflammatory diet. They were impressed by what they found and recommended the approach described in the following pages.

The key foods in the anti-inflammatory diet are antioxidants (see below) and omega 3 fatty acids (see pages 96–7). Calder claims that these substances suppress the production of pro-inflammatory chemicals.

Antioxidants

The recommended anti-inflammatory diet is high in anti-oxidants, the most important nutrients for maintaining good health, reducing inflammation and giving protection during the stress of disease. Antioxidants play a major role in fighting the unstable oxygen atoms known as free radicals, which can run riot around our bodies, destroying cell walls, depleting the cells of energy, and damaging DNA (the self-replicating material that carries genetic information individual to each person). Research has shown that people with higher levels of free radicals are more likely to have ill health than those with lower levels. In some instances, free radicals can even be the cause of disease.

Antioxidants are vitally important because they mop up these destructive free radicals. As a result, the joints are more protected and inflammation reduced. It is even thought that a person who is genetically programmed to develop arthritis can stave off the condition by following an antioxidant-rich diet, as discussed in this chapter.

I should mention here that both cigarette and cigar smoking greatly increases free-radical damage. Indeed, it is known that smokers have low levels of antioxidants in their bodies. An antioxidant-rich diet can reduce free-radical damage, but by far the best option is to give up smoking.

Another happy outcome of a steady intake of antioxidant foods is a longer life. This is because antioxidants secure optimum functioning of each of the millions of cells in our bodies, making them far more productive and preventing their early death.

Fresh fruit and vegetables are the main antioxidant storehouses. They are also present in certain other foods, as discussed in later pages.

Avoid pro-inflammatory foods

Pro-inflammatory foods are known to exacerbate inflammation, increase pain, and heighten your chances of developing chronic conditions.

Foods that can increase inflammation include the following:

- Junk food (also known as 'fast food'). Unhealthy trans-fats and saturated fats are usually used to prepare and process this.
- Saturated fat. This is mostly of animal origin and found in full-fat dairy products (such as cream, cheese, butter and full-fat milk), and processed foods (such as bought cakes, pastries, pies and biscuits). Saturated fat is the most important type

of fat to reduce as it can increase inflammation and pain. Instead of using dairy produce made from animal fats, use oils derived from vegetable, olive, rapeseed or flax. Corn and sunflower oils are high in compounds known as **omega 6 polyunsaturates** which can increase inflammation, and so are best avoided. Any fat on your meat should be trimmed off and you should grill your food instead of frying it. Choose low-fat milk, cream and cheese.

- Processed meats such as luncheon meat, cured hams, paté, salami, hot dogs and sausages. Such foods are not recommended as the processing action can boost the levels of chemicals present such as nitrites, and these are associated with increased inflammation and chronic disease.

- Sugar, such as that found in sweetened cereals, cakes, pies, biscuits, sweets, chocolate, fizzy drinks and that added to cereal and hot drinks. The spikes in blood sugar levels caused by sugar intake are believed by some experts to cause or worsen inflammation. Sugar also has no food value so can be eliminated without loss of nourishment. Get used to sweetening your food by adding raisins, sultanas, honey and maple syrup. If you must use sugar, try to make it muscovado instead of white. Muscovado are the first crude crystals that appear when sugar beet and cane are processed. It is brown and sticky and contains healthy organic acids.

- Experts now think the nightshade family of plants may increase inflammation – these include tomatoes, potatoes, peppers (capsicum) and aubergine (known as eggplant in the USA). The reason for this is that they contain a chemical alkaloid called **solanine** which triggers pain in some people. It seems that not everyone reacts badly to the nightshade family of plants, however. Some friends of mine with arthritis wouldn't dream of eating foods from this family, but others don't react at all to them – while I myself have a problem only with tomatoes. I used to eat a lot of tomato in the form of pasta sauces and chilli. After virtually cutting out tomatoes in the last few months, I have noticed a decrease in my pain levels.

Foods to eat

Eating an anti-inflammatory diet is believed to decrease inflammation and pain, and to improve overall health. It can also help you to achieve the optimum weight for your size.

Fresh fruit and vegetables

Research has indicated that eating a diet high in vitamin C – the most important antioxidant – reduces the risk of developing arthritis. Fresh fruit and vegetables are actually antioxidant 'powerhouses', and the many vitamins, minerals, bioflavonoids and enzymes they contain work together to combat disease and keep the body in good condition. However, vitamin C is rapidly used up in the body by smoking, alcohol consumption, surgery, trauma, stress, exposure to allergens and the use of certain medications.

Brightly coloured fruits and vegetables have the highest antioxidant content. They include apples, oranges, cherries, berries, beetroot, peppers, avocado, sweet potato and leafy green vegetables. These foods are rich in **phytonutrients**, too, these being the chemicals in plants with disease-fighting properties. Moreover, they are high in fibre, which means you feel full quicker (useful if you are attempting to lose weight).

Please note that tomatoes would normally be included in this category, but they are not recommended for people with inflammatory conditions (see page 91 for more information).

Select locally grown, organic fruit and vegetables that are in season – these have the highest nutrient content and the greatest enzyme activity. Organically grown produce may not look as perfect as non-organic, but it is superior. Try to eat it as fresh and as raw as possible. When you have to cook your vegetables, use unsalted (or lightly salted) water and simmer for the minimum length of time. Lightly steaming and stir-frying are healthy alternatives. Scrub your vegetables rather than peel them.

We should all eat five portions of fruit and vegetables a day for optimum health. One portion weighs about 80 grams and is roughly the size of your fist. The following amounts equate to one portion:

- one medium-sized fruit (banana, apple, pear, orange);
- one slice of a large fruit (melon, pineapple, mango);
- two smaller fruits (plums, satsumas, apricots, peaches);
- a dessert bowl full of salad;
- three heaped tablespoonfuls of vegetables;
- three heaped tablespoonfuls of pulses (chickpeas, lentils, beans);
- two to three tablespoonfuls of grapes or berries;
- one tablespoonful of dried fruit;
- one glass (150 ml) of unsweetened fruit or vegetable juice (if you drink two or more glasses of juice, it still only counts as one portion).

Legumes (peas, beans and lentils)

Legumes are rich in protein, which is vital to the bones, joints and all the body systems for growth and maintenance. A deficiency in protein, therefore, can result in more damage to the joints (as well as other areas) than might otherwise occur.

The soya bean is a complete protein, of which there are many derivatives including soya milk, tofu, tempeh, edamame and miso. Tofu, for example, is very versatile and can be used in both savoury and sweet dishes. Soya milk can be used as an alternative to cow's milk.

Seeds

Sunflower, sesame, hemp, linseed (also known as flaxseed) and pumpkin seeds are important for strengthening the immune system and therefore reducing inflammation. They can be eaten as they are as a snack, sprinkled on to salads and cereals, or used in baking. For more flavour they can be lightly roasted and coated with organic soy sauce. Cracked linseed and pumpkin seeds are also highly nutritious, and good for treating constipation. They can be used in baking and sprinkled on to breakfast cereals, over salads, soups and porridge oats.

Nuts

Nuts, too, are intrinsic to strengthening the immune system and so reducing inflammation. All nuts contain vital nutrients, but almonds, cashews, walnuts, Brazils and pecans perhaps offer the greatest array. Eat a wide assortment as snacks, with cereal and in baking. Obviously, if you are allergic to nuts, they must be avoided at all costs.

Fibre

Fibre, in the form of wholegrain foods and wholemeal flours, is rich in complex unrefined carbohydrates, which are excellent for health. Consuming at least three servings of wholegrain foods daily can also help you to achieve your optimum weight (being overweight is a great strain on arthritic joints, as discussed on pages 99–100).

Here are some further tips for eating wholegrains:

- Try to eat a bowl of porridge for breakfast every day, buy oatmeal biscuits and oat cereal bars.
- Use brown rice instead of white.
- Choose wholegrain pasta.
- Choose bean-thread noodles, rice noodles or Japanese noodles such as udon and soba.
- If you can eat wheat, use whole wheat pasta instead of refined white pasta.
- Use wholegrains such as barley in soups and stews.
- Use bulgur wheat in casseroles and stir-fries.
- Make a pilaf with wholegrains such as wild rice, brown rice and barley.
- Substitute half the refined white flour in pancakes, buns and other flour-based recipes for whole wheat or oat flour.
- Use rolled oats or crushed unsweetened wholegrain cereal to bread chicken, fish, veal cutlets and so on.
- Use wholegrain flour or oatmeal when making baked treats.
- Read the ingredient list – the colour of a grain is not an indication of whether or not it is 'whole'.

With the exception of wheat (a common allergen), aim to consume a variety of grains, including oats, rye, barley (generally available as pearl barley), corn, buckwheat, brown rice and mixed grains. Brown rice, millet, buckwheat and maize/corn are all gluten-free and invaluable to people with a gluten allergy.

Note that white pasta and white rice (both of which are highly refined) can trigger or worsen inflammation, so are best eliminated from your diet. If, for some reason, you can't avoid eating them, cook them *al dente*. Your body should then not metabolize them so quickly and you might escape the sudden detrimental rise in your blood sugar levels.

Fats and oils

Fats are the most concentrated sources of energy in our diet, with one gram of fat providing the body with nine calories of energy. They are also a fine source of essential fatty acids (EFAs), which play a large role in reducing inflammation, as mentioned on pages 96–7. As our bodies are unable to manufacture fatty acids, they can only come from our diets. A deficiency in EFAs is linked with muscle tissue wasting, reduced immune-system function, an increase in inflammation and diminished cognitive ability.

There are two distinct types of EFA – one bad, one good:

Saturated fat

Believed to be implicated in the development of both disease and inflammation, saturated fat comes mainly from animal sources and is generally solid at room temperature. Margarine was, for many years, believed to be a healthier choice over butter, but nutritionists have now revised their opinion. This is because some of the fats in the margarine hydrogenation process are changed into trans-fatty acids which the body metabolizes as if they were saturated fatty acids – the same as butter. Butter is a valuable source of oils and vitamin A, but should be used very sparingly. Margarine, on the other hand, is an artificial product containing many additives. It is therefore not recommended.

Unsaturated fat

Also called polyunsaturated or monounsaturated fat, unsaturated fat has a protective effect on the heart and other organs. Omega

3 and omega 6 EFAs both occur naturally in oily fish (mackerel, herring, sardines, tuna, etc.), nuts and seeds, and are usually liquid at room temperature. It is recommended, then, that you eat oily fish at least three times a week and cold-pressed oil (olive, rapeseed and safflower oil) daily, for dressings and in cooking.

It is important to note that the process of *frying* changes the molecular structure of foods, rendering them potentially damaging to the body. If you must fry something, it is best to use a small amount of extra virgin olive oil and cook at a low temperature. Sautéing in a little water or tomato juice can be quite acceptable, otherwise grilling, baking and steaming are alternatives.

I must add a word of warning: never re-heat used oils, for this, too, can be harmful to the body.

It is possible to cut out saturated fats by reading the food label. This should say whether the food in question is 'low fat', 'low in saturated fat', 'medium fat', 'medium in saturated fat', 'high fat', or 'high in saturated fat'. These translate to the following:

- low – less than 3 grams of total fat or 1 gram of saturated fat per 100 grams of food; 'low fat' or 'low in saturated fat' is a good choice;
- medium – between 3 and 20 grams of total fat or between 1 and 5 grams of saturated fat per 100 grams of food; it is recommended that you only eat small amounts of 'medium fat' or 'medium in saturated fat', on an occasional basis;
- high – more than 20 grams of total fat or 5 grams of saturated fat per 100 grams of food; high-fat products should be avoided altogether.

Omega 3 versus omega 6 fatty acids

Although I mentioned above that EFAs are important for reducing inflammation, I must explain the value of a good dietary balance between omega 3 and omega 6 EFAs. Both of these EFAs are beneficial to health – but it's not that simple. The two are metabolically different and have opposing physiological functions. Both are of use in different ways, but only if your diet is balanced approximately 2:1 in favour of omega 3. In other words, double the intake of omega 3 over omega 6 is required. Research has indicated that individuals with a higher balance of omega

3 to omega 6 are less likely to have heart disease, hypertension, arthritis, cancer, other inflammatory conditions and autoimmune disorders. On the other hand, people who consume more omega 6 than omega 3 are likely to have an increased incidence of cardiovascular disease and inflammatory disorders.

Unfortunately, the modern diet has an excess of omega 6 and a shortfall of omega 3, which can cause or worsen inflammation and create problems within the circulatory system. I was actually quite shocked to learn that, in general, most people consume between ten and twenty times more omega 6 than omega 3! As getting the balance of these EFAs is so important, it can be assumed that the majority of people in the Western world need to eat far more omega 3 and cut back on the amount of omega 6 they consume. You don't need to bring your calculator into the kitchen either, you just need to concentrate on including more omega 3 EFAs in your diet.

The top food sources of omega 3 EFAs include fish and seafood (such as fresh tuna, sardines, halibut, shrimp, snapper, cod, salmon and scallops), as well as linseed (also called flaxseed), walnuts, winter squash, olive oil, soy beans, kidney beans and tofu. Linseed and walnuts have the highest omega 3 content of all. They can be sprinkled on to salads, baked potatoes, porridge, muesli and granola.

Omega 3 is now increasingly being added to everyday foods by companies who, luckily, are cashing in on the media hype. To date, these foods include certain types of bread, yoghurt, fruit juice, baked beans and tinned pasta. Look at the list of ingredients before buying.

Eggs

Contrary to long-held opinion, the cholesterol in eggs is not now thought to be a risk factor for health. Eggs contain lecithin, a superb 'biological detergent' capable of breaking down fats so they can be utilized by the body. In addition, lecithin prevents the accumulation of too many acid or alkaline substances in the blood and encourages the transport of nutrients through cell walls. Buy free-range eggs and eat them soft boiled (or soft poached) as a hard yolk will bind the lecithin, rendering it useless as a 'fat-detergent'.

The Food Standards Agency now states that most people don't need to limit their consumption of eggs so long as they are part of a balanced diet.

Red meat

As red meat is high in omega 6 EFAs (see pages 95–7) and often loaded with saturated fat (see page 95), it should be consumed in moderation. Look for organically produced meat as the pesticides, antibiotics and hormones used in animal husbandry is an ongoing health issue. If you can't bear to go without red meat, make your serving no larger or thicker than the palm of your hand, and try not to eat red meat more than two or three times a week.

Unfortunately, reducing your consumption of red meat will lower your protein intake (see page 93 for information on the benefits of protein). You should, therefore, ensure that you eat plenty of other protein-containing foods such as fish, poultry, soya products, cottage cheese, organic live yogurt, nuts, seeds and legumes. Low protein intake causes the body to pull protein from the muscles, resulting in weakness, low energy, low stamina, depression and poor resistance to infection. A person with arthritis who eats a low protein diet risks further joint damage, too.

Here are some suggestions for buying, cooking and eating red meat:

- Choose the leanest cuts of meat you can find. The leanest beef cuts include top loin, top sirloin and shoulder. The leanest pork cuts include pork loin, tenderloin and ham. The leanest lamb cuts are from the shank half of the leg.
- Trim away any visible fat before cooking.
- Grill, roast, poach or boil red meat instead of frying.
- If you must on the odd occasion fry your meat, don't bread it as this adds fat and causes the meat to soak up more fat.
- Choose extra lean minced meat.
- Any fat that arises from cooking should be carefully drained off.
- Ham, sausages, frankfurters, burgers and luncheon meats are processed and contain added sodium (salt). Unless it says 'low sodium content' on the label, they should be avoided.
- As lower-fat processed meats are now available in shops, check out the nutrition facts on the label and choose processed meats with less saturated fat.

Fish

Fish is a nutritious alternative to red meat. It is an excellent source of omega 3 fatty acids, gamma linoleic acid (GLA) and the amino acids our bodies need to build protein. Choose cold water fish, especially oily fish such as sardines, fresh tuna, anchovies, mackerel, trout, salmon, herring (kippers) and pilchards. Try to avoid frying your fish. Poach, grill or bake instead. Also, it is not wise to cover fish in breadcrumbs as this adds more fat and makes the fish soak up additional fat.

Poultry

Poultry such as chicken and turkey contains far less fat than red meat, and is a good source of protein and EFAs, which can help to stave off illness and fight existing disease. It is therefore recommended that you eat chicken or turkey once or twice a week. The leanest poultry choices are boneless chicken breasts and turkey cutlets. Fresh chicken and turkey is usually 'flavour enhanced' by the addition of sodium (salt). Avoid poultry with 'self-basting' on the label as this is an indication of sodium addition. Even better, look for 'organic' and 'free range' on the label.

Arthritis and being overweight

If you have arthritis and are overweight, you are putting an unnecessary burden on your weight-bearing joints (such as the neck, back, hips, knees, ankles and feet). If these joints have already undergone some degree of damage, the additional weight will only serve to accelerate the destructive process.

Joints are under a lot of pressure when we walk – particularly our knee joints which carry five or six times our body weight at each step. This means that even a small weight loss can ease the load considerably. An excess of body fat can also increase inflammation in the body, as was shown in blood tests for inflammation levels after a number of individuals lost weight.

To find out how much weight you need to lose, if any, you can calculate your body mass index (BMI); see Figure 2. This can be done by multiplying your height in metres by itself to give you figure 'A'. Next, divide your weight in kilograms by your figure A – this is your BMI. For most people, the ideal BMI is 20–25.

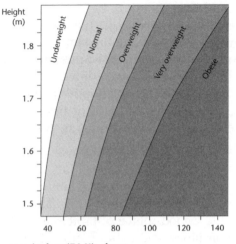

Figure 2 Body mass index (BMI) chart

How do I lose weight?

If you are overweight, the best way to lose weight and keep it off is to make permanent changes to the way you eat. Crash and fad diets are not recommended as they are unsustainable and usually far too limited in the nourishment they provide. As soon as you stop the diet and return to your normal way of eating, you are likely to very quickly put back on all the weight you lost.

Eating a healthy diet is the best way to lose weight. As well as being an anti-inflammatory diet, the diet suggested in this

Here are a few more guidelines for better eating. They should encourage weight loss in people who need to lose weight:

- Avoid invisible fats in cakes, biscuits, etc. Check the label if you are unsure.
- Choose lean cuts of meat.
- Trim any excess fat off your meat.
- Eat more fresh fish and poultry.
- Drink low-fat milk – i.e. skimmed or semi-skimmed.
- Eat low-fat dairy products – i.e. yoghurt, cream and butter.
- Avoid using margarine. If you can't avoid it, choose olive oil based or soya margarine.
- Avoid frying your food. Grill instead.
- Eat plenty of wholegrain bread, cereals, fruit and vegetables.
- Eat healthy snacks such as nuts, seeds, raisins, dried and fresh fruit.

chapter is balanced and good for health. It contains less fat and sugar than might otherwise be eaten – that is, chocolate, sweets, cakes, biscuits, pastries, pies and savoury snacks. It also contains more fruit and vegetables as well as other health-giving foods.

Do I need to take supplements?

Vitamin and mineral supplements are very popular for people with arthritis – but are they of any benefit? Well, many experts recommend them, some people swear by them, and many others claim they make no difference at all. I can only say that if there are shortfalls in particular vitamins and minerals from the foods in your diet, it might be best to take them in supplement form instead.

Some people recommend an array of supplements, which can be very expensive. It is actually best to get the vitamins and minerals you need from food rather than supplements. However, supplements can be invaluable for people who don't like certain foods and/or have severe nutritional deficiencies.

Before taking supplements, bear the following in mind:

- Try to work out which supplements will be of most benefit for your particular problems and find out as much about them as possible.
- Take one type of supplement at a time, so you can best gauge its efficacy.
- Keep a record of how you are feeling on a daily basis so you can assess whether the supplements are having an effect. If you have not improved in any way after three months, stop taking them.
- Inform your doctor of any supplements you are about to take. Check that they will not interact with your prescription medications.
- Report any untoward side effects immediately.
- Purchase from reputable companies for a better product.
- Remember supplements can not cure chronic conditions.

The following vitamins and minerals are thought to be of most benefit to people with arthritis:

Vitamin C. This vitamin is a fine antioxidant, helping to rid the body of the free radicals that are so destructive to the joints. Indeed, a range of studies have shown that people with diets high in vitamin C have significantly less chance of their arthritis progressing. As our bodies are unable to manufacture or store this vitamin, it can only be obtained from our diets – it is largely found in citrus fruits and fresh vegetables. It can also be acquired in supplement form. Avoid taking a large dose in the morning, however, as your body will simply flush out what it doesn't immediately need. It is best to take a three-times-a-day supplement, and even better to eat plenty of foods that are rich in vitamin C. About 60 mg of vitamin C is the recommended daily allowance (RDA), but people with arthritis require 200–300 mg. Note that to consume in excess of 500 mg daily can cause digestive problems and interfere with the absorption of other nutrients.

Vitamin D. Because ultraviolet light converts the precursors of this antioxidant vitamin into a form the body can use, it can be obtained by merely standing in the sun. Many people with arthritis are deficient in vitamin D – and since vitamin D protects the bones and joints, someone with arthritis can be prone to developing thin and brittle bones (osteoporosis). To ensure that your bones and joints don't deteriorate too much, get 10–15 minutes of exposure to sunlight about three times a week, eat foods that are rich in vitamin D such as D-fortified milk, cheese, ice cream, butter and yoghurt. Check the label to see whether your selected item is indeed fortified before buying it. If you don't get to see much sunshine or can't tolerate dairy products, it may be best to take vitamin D supplements. Avoid taking high doses, though, as excess amounts are stored in the body and can become toxic to the soft tissues of the heart and kidneys. Follow the label dosage instructions.

Vitamin E. This antioxidant vitamin is not so strong as vitamins C and D, but it still helps to protect the joints and other parts from the ravages of free radicals. It can be obtained by cooking with soybean oil or canola oil. It is also present in fish, avocados, wheatgerm, nuts, pumpkin seeds and sunflower seeds, and in smaller amounts in cabbage, asparagus and Brussels sprouts. If you don't think you obtain enough vitamin E from food sources, you might want to try taking fish oil capsules and follow the dosage instructions.

B vitamins. Various studies have shown that most people don't consume enough of the B vitamins, especially women. There is evidence that the inflammatory process uses up a lot of the B vitamins present in the body, so it is necessary to eat a lot of foods rich in this group. Spinach, fortified cereal, tuna, sardines and fortified cottage cheese contain varying amounts of the B vitamins. To ensure that you are obtaining enough, it may be best to take them in supplement form as well. Follow the label dosage instructions.

Calcium. As more than 90 per cent of calcium in the body is stored in the bones, it is of obvious importance in arthritis – yet most people have a shortfall of this mineral, which can lead to osteoporosis. Good food sources of calcium are dairy products, cauliflower, cabbage, kale, broccoli,

Brussels sprouts, turnip and fish that have edible bones – such as sardines. As vitamin D boosts the body's absorption of calcium, you can get the optimum benefit by taking the two together – that is, in D-fortified milk. If you think you need more calcium, you might like to try supplementation, following the label dosage instructions. You could also ask your doctor to send you for regular bone density scans. If you are diagnosed with osteoporosis, you will be prescribed an excellent supplement regime of calcium and vitamin D. I have used this therapy for the last three years and my osteoporosis is now markedly improved, as shown in my scans.

Magnesium. Calcium works to tighten and constrict bodily tissues, including the bones, whereas its 'sister' mineral, magnesium, exerts a relaxing effect. In fact, calcium and magnesium work together to ensure proper muscle contraction/relaxation, and the building of muscle fibres and connective tissues. Magnesium deficiency is as common as that of calcium, however – and, due to the precarious balance between these two associated minerals, deficiency can also be caused by excessive calcium supplementation. Junk foods are frequently low in magnesium, and processed bran added to a poor diet can render magnesium useless. Good food sources include wholegrains, leafy green vegetables, nuts (especially almonds and cashews), seeds, legumes, low-fat tofu and soy products, vegetables (especially broccoli and sweetcorn), bananas and apricots. Follow the dosage instructions. Note that if you take high doses of magnesium, it can become toxic to the body. It can also interact with other medications. Therefore if you wish to take magnesium, it is best to discuss it with your doctor. Magnesium supplementation is particularly recommended for treating fibromyalgia.

Selenium. This major antioxidant protects cells from the toxic effects of free radicals and, in so doing, boosts the immune system. It is therefore of benefit for people with inflammatory conditions. Good food sources are tuna, salmon, shrimp, garlic, sunflower seeds, Brazil nuts and wheat breads. As the body does not require high levels of this mineral, it is best taken as part of a multivitamin supplement.

Zinc. Some studies have found that zinc – an important antioxidant – reduces morning stiffness and joint inflammation. People with RA are often deficient in zinc. Vegetarians may also have a shortfall, with the high grain content of their diets binding the zinc and rendering it useless. Zinc should be accompanied by copper in a ratio of 10–15 mg of zinc to 1 mg of copper, to prevent a possible copper imbalance. If you think you are deficient in zinc and wish to take a supplement, it is best as part of a multivitamin preparation. Good food sources are the herb licorice, oysters, lean meats, liver, wheatgerm, pumpkin seeds, sunflower seeds and ginseng.

7

Activity and exercise

Being active and following a gentle daily exercise programme is an important part of a successful treatment regime for arthritis. It is vital in improving muscle tone, joint mobility and general stamina, all of which can be impaired in arthritis. Activity and exercise can also halt the progressive deterioration of your condition that might otherwise occur. If, however, your arthritis is so severe that you require help in order to accomplish even the smallest of tasks, embarking upon an exercise regime is likely to be the last thing on your mind. Don't panic at the thought of activity and exercise, though. You are likely to be able to cope comfortably with at least one form of exercise, even if it means embarking upon it in a very small way. In time, as you gain in strength and flexibility, you should be able to extend your chosen exercise programme and perhaps start going to the local swimming pool or taking a short daily walk.

Muscle-strengthening exercises can help to build up your muscles, which in turn provide better support for the joints and so reduce the risk of a joint giving way. Stronger muscles around the knees and ankles are usually of particular benefit as these two areas can be prone to developing osteoarthritis. See page 118 for more information on strengthening exercises.

Being physically active

People who are able to remain physically active – and who can incorporate an exercise regime into their daily lives – stand the best chance of making improvements. Activity and exercises also reduce the risk of future health problems developing. If you are still able to live a fairly active life, it is important that you keep up your levels of activity, gradually introducing an exercise plan into your daily routine (as discussed in this chapter). Listening to your body will help you to judge whether or not you have overdone the activity/exercise on a particular day and you'll learn from that.

Regular exercise can help you to manage arthritis in the following ways:

- It can help to reduce pain levels.
- It can increase strength, mobility and range of movement.
- It helps to maintain your sense of independence.
- It reduces stress levels.
- It improves kidney function.
- It can help to maintain a healthy weight.
- It aids weight loss in people who are overweight.
- It can help to improve posture.

Physiotherapy

If your stiffness and pain levels mean you struggle to remain active or have been forced to become immobile for large chunks of the day, your doctor or rheumatologist will probably refer you for physiotherapy – a treatment with a major role in managing arthritis. Chartered physiotherapists are usually based in hospital departments and health centres. They usually work alone, but some operate within a team of healthcare professionals in which case you may be seen in a group session. Here you will meet people with similar problems and learn exercises and so on together.

If your doctor or rheumatologist doesn't automatically refer you for physiotherapy, you can always ask to be referred. You could also see a physiotherapist privately by looking for details in *Yellow Pages* or your local *Thomson Directory*. Alternatively, you can contact the Organisation of Chartered Physiotherapists in Private Practice. It is important to check that a physiotherapist has the letters MCSP after his or her name, which means he or she has completed a high standard of training.

Physiotherapists are taught to understand the complexities of the human body and the way it moves. They are accustomed to working with people with limited mobility – that is, as a result of injury, arthritis or another condition. Their assessment begins with observing your gait as you walk and looking for any movement difficulties or joint deformities. They ask questions about your pain, stiffness and so on, then offer you advice on such things as how to look after vulnerable joints, how to improve your posture, and walking aids. You may also be offered a course of hydrotherapy in a special heated pool.

It is usual to have six physiotherapy sessions during which a personalized treatment plan is put into operation. Their plan may include:

- designing an exercise programme for you to mobilize your joints and strengthen the supporting muscles (note that when the physiotherapy sessions are finished, the exercise programme should be carried out at home on a long-term basis);
- teaching you relaxation techniques, the aim being to reduce the muscle tension that can make arthritis feel worse;
- showing you how to improve your posture and find ways of performing tasks that exert the least strain on your joints (see Chapter 8);
- massaging areas of your body that are affected by arthritis in order to release any tension knots that are adding to your pain;
- using pain relief techniques, such as electrotherapy; this is where electric currents are passed through your body to stimulate the nerves and muscles in areas that may feel numb or that have not been used for a long time;
- using TENS (transcutaneous electrical nerve stimulation) to provide pain relief. Electrodes are applied to the skin over the painful areas and an electrical impulse delivered through them from a small, portable device you can clip to your belt or waistband. The impulses delivered from the TENS machine are intended to block the pain signals coming from underlying nerves. TENS machines are available for purchase from some hospitals, health centres and pharmacies. They should be tried out on different frequencies to find out which one works best for you.

Occupational therapy (OT)

Joints that are inflamed or damaged by arthritis need to be protected and looked after. Keeping as healthy and fit as possible is part of this, as is maintaining a normal weight. It's also important to avoid straining your joints by repetitive activity and awkward posture. You should, therefore, give a lot of thought as to how you bend, lift and carry things, particularly if you find certain everyday tasks like dressing, washing, cooking and cleaning difficult to do (see Chapter 8 for details of how to improve your posture in a variety of situations).

Your local OT department can offer invaluable advice regarding these things, too. They can also help to organize your home and working environment to your best advantage. You may be loaned certain useful equipment – usually the more expensive apparatus – and told where you can buy further items. For example, long-handled 'reachers' are very useful, as are 'shoppers' (on wheels), 'hands-free' telephones, electric can openers, jar openers that grip, electric carving knives, juicers and food processors. OT departments also loan out such things as support splints to protect inflamed joints.

Your doctor or physiotherapist may refer you to the OT department at your local hospital. The job of an occupational therapist is to find ways to keep people as independent as possible despite their condition. OT departments achieve this by offering advice on:

- coping with everyday tasks such as washing, dressing and cooking;
- adapting your home, making it more accessible so you can function more easily;
- how best to enjoy leisure activities;
- cars, wheelchairs and the best ways to get around;
- any benefits to which you may be entitled;
- suitable employment.

If your details have been passed on to your local OT department, someone from there is likely to want to visit you at home to offer advice (as mentioned above) and to assess whether certain adaptations would make life easier for you. If your doctor or rheumatologist has not yet referred you to an OT department, you can ask social services (look in the phone book under the name of your local authority) for an assessment of your requirements under the NHS and Community Care Act 1990.

Disability employment advisers (DEAs)

You also have the option of seeing a disability employment adviser (DEA), based at your local Jobcentre Plus. These people offer professional advice and support to disabled people who are well enough to move from benefits on to working, and to others who need to find a less physically demanding job. They also inform you of your rights and options within the work environment. If necessary, DEAs offer practical help with things such as compiling your CV, filling out application forms, and giving tips on interview techniques.

People who have previously given up work due to their arthritis may be offered a new lease of life in the form of retraining, further education or voluntary work. The DEA will ensure, too, that the Disability Discrimination Act (DDA) is observed by employers at all times. This means that, if possible, an employer should make it easier for a person with mobility problems to access their place of employment, such as by relocating them to the ground floor of the building or to a more reachable work station. An employer would also be expected, under the DDA, to retrain you in a less taxing job.

Of course, you must be sure to tell your employer that you have arthritis before the DDA can protect you.

The Access to Work programme

The Access to Work programme is a government scheme aimed at assisting disabled people to find answers to problems that have deterred them from finding or keeping a job. For example, advisers on the scheme can provide specialized equipment or make any necessary adaptations to your workplace, once this has been agreed by all parties involved. In some cases, they can even help you to get to and from work, organizing a free taxi if you are unable to drive or take the bus or train. For further information, contact your local Jobcentre Plus.

The right type of exercise

Doing the right type of exercise regularly can help people with arthritis to manage the condition. It is also fundamental to general improvement. So what exactly do I mean by 'the right type of exercise', I can almost hear you say! I mean:

- carrying out a daily exercise programme tailored to your own particular needs – that is, if you have arthritis in your knees, you should choose exercises aimed at strengthening the muscles, tendons and ligaments (soft tissues) around the knee; likewise, if you have arthritis in your hips, you should choose exercises aimed at building up the soft tissues in your hip, lower back and thigh muscles;
- doing general exercises aimed at building up your strength, stamina and range of movement; because arthritis doesn't develop overnight, performing a 'generalized routine' can help to slow down the progress of the condition in other areas of your body;
- engaging in aerobic exercise on a regular basis; the exercise you choose should be appropriate to your strength and capability – for example, walking, swimming, cycling or ball games such as tennis or badminton.

Note that being active and performing a daily exercise routine can not only increase your strength, stamina and range of movement, it can also help you to maintain a healthy weight, improve your posture, and reduce your chances of developing osteoporosis. Perhaps the real key to success, though, is being realistic about the amount of exercise/activity you can cope with at a particular time. Expecting to do exercise of some sort for an hour each day may be far too much, especially on those days when the stiffness and pain are worse than usual. Indeed, it may quickly end up in failure, provoking feelings of uselessness and making you less likely to do exercise in the future.

I remember that in the early days of my fibromyalgia (a type of arthritis, as mentioned on pages 26–30), I was bed-bound and could not look after myself in any way. When my rheumatologist assured me that embarking on a regular careful exercise regime would give me my best chance of improvement, I thought he was mad, and that he clearly had no notion of how much pain I was in. My doctor and pain specialist gave me the very same advice, though, and I finally accepted that I must take exercise seriously.

I began by sitting on my supportive bedside chair for a few minutes to carry out a simple stretching exercise twice daily. My neck and shoulders were so painful at that time that I was unable put my hands on top of my head, so I simply raised them as far as they would comfortably go. Within a few weeks the action became a little easier and soon I was stretching my arms straight up, high into the air. In the coming months, I was able to add further stretching exercises to my repertoire and the result was a noticeable improvement in my overall state.

When I was diagnosed with osteoarthritis in my spine (it had most likely been developing over several years), I knew it was time to try adding further movements to my repertoire and increasing the repetitions. If my body could cope with the extra activity, it would be for the good. I did overdo the exercise at times, and it invariably set me back for a while. However, I tried to view the setbacks as 'learning experiences', which (most of the time) stopped me from feeling angry and disappointed. I'm sure that extra activity is partly what has allowed me to avoid further deterioration, and I certainly have far fewer arthritis flare-ups than I could ever have envisaged when I was first diagnosed.

It is always wise to assess your condition before carrying out exercise of any kind. If your symptoms are worse than usual – that is, during a flare-up – it is probably best to do a few very gentle stretches at regular intervals throughout the day to prevent your joints from stiffening further. Between the stretches, take it easy to allow the inflammation to calm down. Make sure that you resume your exercise regime as soon as your body allows; always 'listen to your body' and never force a painful joint. If the pain in your hip is worse than ever on one particular day and it's a choice between exercising (perhaps in the form of intermittent stretches) and doing the vacuuming, you really need to choose the stretches. I know it's hard asking others to do things for you, but if you explain that you are now following a special regime that should help to improve your condition, they will hopefully understand. Alternatively, why not put up with a bit of dust and clutter for a few months, or for however long it takes for the inflammation to calm down? Occasional setbacks are only to be expected when you first embark on an exercise programme, but in the long term, improvement will almost certainly come.

Can older people exercise?

You may wonder whether older people with conditions such as high blood pressure can safely exercise. The answer is a resounding 'yes', so long as you get the go-ahead from your doctor, too. Regular exercise is known to have an energizing effect; it promotes weight loss; reduces stress levels; helps to normalize blood pressure; aids in conditioning the heart muscle; and helps to maintain mobility in the joints.

Planning your exercise regime

It is important to use caution when choosing which exercises to include in your regime. As you read through the exercise possibilities in this chapter, mark the ones you think you can easily do. Keeping in mind your current condition, pick out a few you think you could do from tomorrow, with the aim of adding more to your regime as you improve. Remember that it's not wise to throw yourself straight into a challenging routine. In fact, as a strenuous exercise can cause further pain and joint deterioration, it is best to keep to a moderate routine.

Warm-up exercises

The immobility imposed upon some people with arthritis causes certain muscle groups to be tight and very stiff. Over-stretching these muscles can therefore really hurt and is often the cause of delayed pain. It is essential, therefore, that you do warm-up exercises at the start of your routine.

The warm-up exercises you choose should depend on your fitness levels and particular limitations. For instance, if your arthritis is quite severe and you are out of condition, you need to formulate a gentle programme with basic exercises. It is important to remember that one or two repetitions of several exercises is generally better than several repetitions of only one or two exercises. If you feel you are starting to struggle during your routine, stop immediately and relax. It is far safer to break up one exercise session into two (or even three) parts, completing the full programme later in the day if you still feel up to it.

Stretching exercises

If, after finishing your warm-ups, you think you can carry on, try to do one or two of the easier stretching exercises. You will know by your body's reaction the following day whether your chosen exercises were over-ambitious or whether you allowed insufficient resting time for your body to recover. If your symptoms are definitely worse after doing the exercises, take it easy for a few days then recommence your routine with the most basic of exercises. And make sure you relax afterwards. Ideally, when you finish your exercise routine, you should feel as if you could have done more. Bear in mind that you may be able to do the exercises that you had to drop when your joints and soft tissues are stronger.

Note: Never skip warm-ups in favour of more vigorous exercise.

Mobility exercises

Mobility exercises are the mainstay of every exercise programme as they help to maintain strength, flexibility and range of movement. Many people with arthritis become less active because of the pain and the fear of making themselves worse, but this results in muscle wasting and weaker joints. Mobility exercises, however, can strengthen the muscles and make the joints more flexible, enabling you to walk, swim, climb stairs and so on more easily.

Mobility exercises involve moving the joints through their comfortable range, then easing them a tiny bit further. Movements should be smooth and continuous, performed while your body is in a relaxed state – exercising when tense can cause more harm than good. Keep your back straight, your bottom tucked in, and your stomach flattened as you perform your routine. Stand with your legs slightly apart.

Shoulders

Letting your arms hang loose, slowly circle your shoulders backwards. Repeat the exercise between two and ten times, depending on your condition. Now slowly circle your shoulders forwards and repeat for another two to ten times, as appropriate.

Neck

1 Making sure you are standing up straight, slowly turn your head to the left – as far as it will comfortably go – then hold for a count of two. Return to the centre and repeat the exercise between two and ten times. Now turn your head to the right, holding for a count of two before returning to centre. Repeat between two and ten times.

2 Tucking in your chin, tilt your head down and hold for a count of two. Repeat between two and ten times. Again tucking in your chin, tilt your head upwards, but not so far that it virtually sits on your shoulders, and hold for a count of two. Repeat between two and ten times.

Spine

1 Placing your hands on your hips to help support your lower back, slowly tilt your upper body to the left and hold for a count of two. Return to the centre, then repeat between two and ten times. Now tilt to the right and return to the centre. Repeat between two and ten times (see Figure 3).

2 Keeping your lower back static, gently, in a flowing rather than fast movement, swing your arms and upper body to the left as far as it will comfortably go, then return to the centre. Repeat between two and ten times. Now swing your arms and upper body to the right and return to the centre. Repeat between two and ten times.

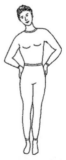

Figure 3 Spine mobility exercise

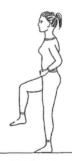

Figure 4 Hips and knees mobility exercise

Hips and knees

With your body upright, move your hips by lifting your left knee upwards, as far as is comfortable. Hold for a count of two, then lower. Now raise your right knee and hold for a count of two before lowering. Repeat between two and ten times (see Figure 4 on the previous page).

Ankles

With your supporting leg slightly bent, place your left heel on the floor in front of you. Lift up your left foot and then place your left toes on the floor. Repeat between two and ten times. Now duplicate the exercise and number of repetitions with the right foot (see Figures 5(a) and (b)).

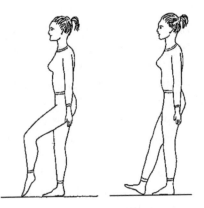

Figures 5(a) and (b) Ankle mobility exercises

Pulse-raising activities

Pulse-raising activities such as walking around the room are still part of your warm-up routine. Before embarking on stretches, it is best to warm your muscles further in this way.

Stretching exercises

The muscles, already becoming warm and flexible, will relax further when mobility and pulse-raising activities are followed by short stretches. Stretches prepare them for the more challenging movements that may follow, if you are up to it. These exercises have been devised with the help of the Health Education Authority.

Again, it is up to you to decide which ones you think you are capable of performing.

Calves

1 Stand with your arms outstretched, your palms against a wall. Keeping your left foot on the floor, bend your left knee and stretch your right leg out behind you. Press the heel of your right foot into the floor until you feel a gentle stretch in your leg muscles. Now change legs. Repeat between two and ten times (see Figure 6).

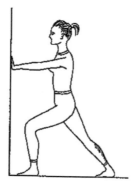

Figure 6 Stretching exercise for the calves

2 Standing with your feet slightly apart, raise both heels off the floor so that you are on your toes. Repeat between two and ten times. As your calf muscles strengthen, you should be able to stay on your toes for longer periods of time. This exercise also helps your balance.

Fronts of the thighs

Using a chair or wall for support, stand with your left leg in front of your right, both knees bent, your right heel off the floor. Tuck in your bottom, and move your hips forwards until you feel a gentle stretch in the front of your right thigh. Now change over legs. Repeat between two and ten times (see Figure 7).

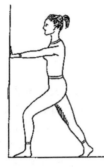

Figure 7 Stretching exercise for the fronts of the thighs

Backs of the thighs

Stand with your legs slightly bent, with your left leg about 20 cm (8 in) in front of your right leg. Keeping your back straight, place both hands on your hips and lean forward a little. Now straighten your left leg, tilting your bottom back until you feel a gentle stretch in the back of your left thigh. Now change over legs. Repeat between two and ten times (see Figure 8).

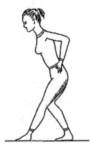

Figure 8 Stretching exercise for the backs of the thighs

Inner thighs

Spreading your legs slightly, your hips facing forwards and with your back straight, bend your left leg and, keeping the right leg straight, move it slowly sideways until you feel a gentle stretch along your inner thigh. Then gently move to the right, bending your right leg as you straighten the left (see Figure 9).

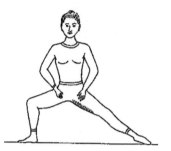

Figure 9 Stretching exercise for the inner thigh

Chest

Keeping your back straight, your knees slightly bent and your pelvis tucked under, place your arms as far behind your lower back as you can and with your hands resting gently on your lower back. Now move your shoulders and elbows back until you feel a gentle stretch in your chest (see Figure 10).

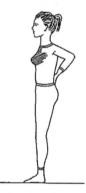

Figure 10 Stretching exercise for the chest

Back of the upper arms

With your knees slightly bent, your back straight and your pelvis tucked under, raise your left arm and bend it so that your hand drops behind your neck and upper back. Using your right hand, apply slight pressure backwards and downwards on your left elbow, until you feel a gentle stretch (see Figure 11).

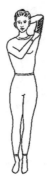

Figure 11 Stretching exercise for the back of the upper arms

Strengthening exercises

The following exercises will build and strengthen your muscles, thus making them more able to protect and support your joints. They should also help to increase your stamina. Remember to incorporate small pauses between repetitions and focus on staying relaxed. Instead of holding your breath on each muscle contraction, it is important to exhale. This allows more blood to flow to the working area.

Thighs

1 Lean back against a wall, your feet 30 cm (12 in) away from the base of the wall. Adopting correct posture, slowly squat down, keeping your heels on the ground. (Don't go too far down at first.) Now slowly straighten your legs. Repeat between two and ten times, lowering yourself further as, over time, your muscles strengthen.
2 Holding on to a sturdy chair and keeping your back 'tall', bend and then slowly straighten both legs, keeping your heels on the floor. Repeat the exercise between two and ten times (see Figure 12).

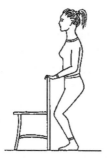

Figure 12 Strengthening exercise for the thighs

3 Sit in a chair and push your knees together, tightening your thigh muscles as you do so. Hold for a few seconds. Repeat between two and ten times.

Upper back

Lie face down on the floor, hands by your side (not on the floor), and keeping your legs straight and tightening your stomach and back muscles, gently raise your head and shoulders. Hold for a count of two, then lower. Repeat between two and ten times (see Figure 13).

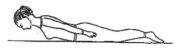

Figure 13 Strengthening exercise for the upper back

Lower back

Lie on your back, using a small rolled-up cloth or towel to support your neck, then bend your knees, keeping your feet on the floor. Lift first your left leg gently behind the knee, pulling it towards your chest until you feel a gentle pull in your bottom and lower back. Repeat with the right leg. Now pull both legs up together. Repeat each exercise between two and ten times (see Figure 14).

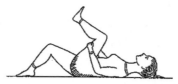

Figure 14 Strengthening exercise for the lower back

Abdomen

1 Lie on your back, using a small rolled-up cloth or towel to support your neck. Bend your knees, keeping your feet flat on the floor. Now tighten your abdominal muscles, tuck your chin in a little towards your chest and raise your head and shoulders, reaching with your arms towards your knees. Remember to keep your lower back pressed down on the floor (see Figure 15).

2 If you are not fit enough to perform sit-ups, the following exercise is just as effective. Lie on your back, using a small rolled-up cloth or towel to support your neck. Pull in your stomach muscles and try to flatten your spine against the floor. Hold for a count of two, then release. Repeat between two and ten times.

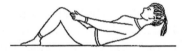

Figure 15 Strengthening exercise for the abdomen

Arms

Place your left hand on your chest and then press for a few seconds. Do the same with your right arm. Repeat between two and ten times.

Push-ups

Stand with your hands flat against a wall, your body straight. Carefully lower your body towards the wall, then slowly push away. Repeat two to ten times. At first, stand quite near the wall, then try moving further away as you become stronger (see Figures 16(a) and (b)).

Using small weights

Lifting weights is a great way to increase muscular strength and improve overall physical fitness. You may wish to use the type that

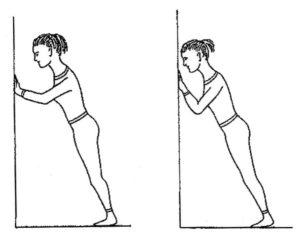

Figures 16(a) and (b) Push-ups

fasten with Velcro around your wrists and ankles and are available from most sports shops. Weights of 225 grams (8 ounces) each slip into small pockets sewn into the band. Start by using one weight only and remember to breathe out as a muscle contracts.

1 With the weights around your wrists, stand with your feet slightly apart. Making sure that only your upper body moves, turn carefully to the left, swinging both arms gently as you move. Repeat two or three times. Now perform the same exercise and number of repetitions, but this time swing your body and arms to the right. Ensure that the movements are steady and fluid, and not too fast.

2 Keeping your left elbow close to your waist, slowly raise your left forearm so it almost touches your shoulder. Lower the forearm until it is at right angles with your upper arm, then slowly raise it again. Now repeat the exercise with your right arm, again ensuring your movements are steady and continuous.

3 Bending your left arm, bringing your hand up until your wrist is level with your shoulder, reach your hand upwards until your elbow is level with your shoulder. Bring it straight

back down to the original position. Repeat once more, then do the same with your right arm.

As you gain in strength and flexibility you may, first, be able to increase the number of repetitions you do and, second, add to the weight you lift. If you have an ongoing pain condition and your pain levels are higher than normal the next day, it is recommended that you postpone these exercises until you feel stronger.

Aerobic exercise

Aerobic exercise increases muscle temperature which makes the soft tissues relax. It ensures they receive more oxygen and that waste products are removed more efficiently – the result being substantial relief from stiffness and pain. Regular aerobic activity also increases your stamina levels and helps you to lose weight. Ideally, to get the most benefit, you should aim to carry out aerobic exercise three to four times a week, for 20–30 minutes. This may be far too much for some people with arthritis. You may be surprised, though, at your progress if you take care to start slowly and very gradually build up your time. Remember not to push yourself unnecessarily during aerobic exercise. A little is better than none at all.

Note: Check with your doctor before going ahead with aerobic exercise.

Walking

Ensure you choose an aerobic exercise you enjoy and one that is within your physical – and practical – scope. Walking is good. It is a weight-bearing activity that increases mobility, strength, stamina and helps protect against osteoporosis (thinning bones). If walking is difficult or you are very out of condition, you may just want to walk to the nearest lamp post and back on your first day. On the second and third days, you could try to repeat that. On the fourth day, you could try walking halfway to the second lamp post, on the fifth and sixth days to repeat that, on the seventh all the way to the second lamp post, on the eighth and ninth days to repeat that, and so on.

Of course, many people with arthritis are barely able to walk due to pain in their knees, hips, ankles or feet. However, most have periods of remission when the pain is not too dire, and it is at such times that they should try very carefully to take a short walk every day – even if it's only around their garden, with the help of one or two walking sticks – and building up very gradually so as not to cause a flare-up. You may surprise yourself at how far you can actually walk, after increasing the distance over several weeks.

Unfortunately, walking outdoors is not always practical in the UK climate. An electrically operated treadmill can be an excellent investment, giving you the freedom to walk whenever you wish. Also, as a treadmill offers continuous level walking, people with arthritis can walk for far greater distances than they could hope to on the variable terrain outdoors. Treadmill walking can be made less monotonous by positioning the machine near to a shelf so you can read a book or magazine at the same time. Another alternative is to pass the time by listening to your favourite music or podcasts on an iPod or MP3 player.

Stepping

If you think 'stepping' is an option for you, start with a small step such as a thick book or maybe a catalogue or telephone directory. Make sure it is placed securely against a bottom stair to keep it steady and give you room to move. After two or three weeks, you may be able to use the bottom stair itself. Place first your left foot, then your right one, on the book or step. Now step backwards with first your left foot, then your right. Repeat between two and ten times, then alternate your feet, placing on the step first your right foot, then your left. If you can possibly build up to ten minutes of stepping without causing a flare-up – which is achievable if you are slow and enormously careful – it will greatly boost your agility.

Swimming

Swimming is a useful activity for people who are unable to walk far, cycle or use 'stepping'. Indeed, a pool heated to around

34°C (93°F) allows you to exercise without the risk of injury associated with most other forms of aerobic activity. It works all the joints and muscles in the body without causing undue stress. Moreover, the pressure of the water causes the chest to expand, encouraging deeper breathing and increased oxygen intake. Try to swim once or twice a week, gradually building up your time to one hour per session. If you are unable to swim laps, try simple kicking, treading water or 'slow' running through the water.

Swimming is only recommended if you enjoy the activity and live fairly close to a heated swimming pool. If the baths are a good distance away, you are liable to attend less and less until you eventually give up, which can provoke feelings of failure.

Aqua-aerobics

Rather than exercising alone in the swimming baths, you may wish to join an aqua-aerobics class. Aqua-aerobics can bring you into contact with those who have similar health problems, enabling you to help and support one another. The class teacher will ensure that you exercise properly for maximum benefit.

Because water supports your body as you exercise – when you are submerged to the neck, you bear only about a tenth of your body weight – the shock factor is removed. Thus your muscles are conditioned with the minimum of discomfort. Once again, exercising in a pool heated to around 34°C (93°F) is best as this soothes the joints, relieves stiffness and encourages better blood circulation.

Most public swimming baths run aqua-aerobics sessions, some of which are graded according to ability. As with all forms of exercise, aqua-aerobics are only truly beneficial when performed on a regular basis.

Cycling

Whether you use an exercise bike or do actual cycling outside, this provides a good cardiovascular workout. However, caution must rule if you have arthritis, for although cycling is classed as a non-weight-bearing exercise, the action of pedalling can exert strain on your knees, ankles and hips, maybe provoking a flare-up after the first attempt. Also, owing to the continuous motion, your legs have no opportunity to rest as they would with most other types of exercise. A small hard seat and handlebars set too far forward can be a problem, too.

If your arthritis is mild or in areas of the body that would not be affected by cycling, it is best to start by pedalling very slowly with the tension set low – this makes it easier to build up momentum. Limit your sessions to two or three minutes at first. If you don't experience flare-ups, you may in time be able to cycle for 20 to 30 minutes.

Cooling-down exercises

Cooling down your muscles after exercise is just as important as warming them up beforehand. You can do this by repeating your choice of warm-up exercises for about five minutes.

Getting started on your routine

So, have you checked with your doctor and made your choices? Have you selected the easier exercises with which you plan to start your routine? If so, you should now read the following recommendations. They should help to get you started with the minimum of discomfort.

- Relieve morning stiffness by taking a warm shower shortly after waking.
- Eat a light breakfast to boost your energy levels – don't exercise after a heavy meal.
- Set aside sufficient time to perform your routine – don't be tempted to rush.
- If possible, exercise after your light breakfast, when you are least tired and before your pain levels start to rise.
- Ensure that you are dressed in loose, comfortable clothing and good, supportive trainers.
- Exercise in a warm place, out of draughts.

- Start slowly and carefully. Be sure only to perform two or three repetitions of your chosen exercises. People with milder symptoms will be able to build up to ten repetitions sooner than people with severe symptoms.
- Movements should be kept within your range. If you know that raising your arms past a certain point gives rise to pain in your shoulder, make sure you don't go past that level. You should be able to extend your range with time.
- As you exercise, keep checking your posture. When you allow your head and shoulders to droop, your back to slouch, you put added strain on your muscles. They then burn more energy, causing additional pain and fatigue.
- Take care that you don't involuntarily hold your breath when exercising. Breathe deeply and evenly, breathing out on the effort, when your muscles are contracting.
- Try to visualize the muscle group being exercised. This should prevent other muscle groups accidentally being worked.
- Ensure that you pause between repetitions. As there is a slight delay between muscle contraction and relaxation, contracting a muscle without pausing means you do so when the muscle is already contracted. This causes a build-up of lactic acid in the area concerned, which, in turn, causes stiffness and pain.
- After exercising, it is important to allow time for recovery before attempting further activity. Don't berate yourself if your pain levels are high afterwards. Get some extra rest, then begin a toned-down version of the routine when you are able.
- When you finish you should feel as if you could have done more.
- Don't try to make up for days when you weren't able to do much. Set your limit at the start of each session and stick to it.

8

Posture

How often were we told when we were young, 'Sit up straight', 'Don't round your shoulders' and 'Don't slouch'? But slouching felt comfortable – and still does. In truth, though, it tires the muscles and puts stress on the joints.

Our backs consist of numerous internal and external muscles, all of which must be equally balanced in order to keep the lower back and pelvic regions correctly aligned. It's important to avoid activities that cause a shift in this alignment or we risk incurring further muscle pain and joint problems.

Basic postural recommendations

Here are some basic postural recommendations to help protect your body:

- When standing, ensure that your head is positioned over your shoulders (that is, not drooping forward) and that your body is positioned directly over your feet.
- Try, at all times, to retain the slight hollow in the middle region of your back. When you are either static or performing an activity, your back should take on the form of an elongated 'S'. Using a lumbar support will encourage correct sitting posture.
- Stay relaxed. Maintaining correct posture does not mean tensing your muscles.
- Avoid slouching forward or leaning backwards.
- Avoid twisting.
- Always have your work or other activity close to you so you are not straining forward.
- Rather than leaning to pick something up off the floor, keep your back straight and bend your knees, allowing your larger leg muscles to take the strain.

- Always seek the least physically stressful approach to an activity.
- Invest in energy-saving devices. Long-handled 'grabbers' are useful, as are 'shoppers' (on wheels), 'hands-free' telephones, electric can openers, electric carving knives, and food processors.
- Be as mobile as possible. Maintaining one position for an extended period aggravates the muscles. Keep stretching and shifting your position.
- Alternate work with rest periods.
- As soon as your pain levels begin to rise, stop what you are doing and consider your options. These may include getting help, taking a break, or cancelling the activity altogether.

Advice for specific activities

The following recommendations take account of both general and housework-oriented activities. Before undertaking any activity you must first assess whether you are physically up to it. Try not to take chances, and don't be afraid to delegate. Asking for help does not indicate weakness. It takes guts, and is an essential part of coping.

Sitting for long periods

There may be times when you need to sit for long periods – for example, waiting to see the doctor/dentist, watching a play/film, or at a family gathering. This can put a lot of stress on the joints and soft tissues in the back and hips, so here are some tips:

- Sit, if possible, in a chair that supports your entire back. Chairs that look comfortable are not necessarily the most supportive. Your chosen chair should have adequate lumbar support and armrests – and should seat you higher than a standard armchair. The added height makes it easier for you to stand up.
- Orthopaedic 'high chairs' can these days be purchased from larger furniture retailers, as well as from specialist outlets. If

you are not in your own home, choose the best chair available to sit in – if necessary, politely asking another person if they would mind very much vacating the best seat. (You should always briefly explain why you need a supportive chair.)

- Ensure you always adopt the correct sitting posture. Your bottom should be tucked well into the back of the seat, your spine supported by the back of the chair. Your head should sit directly on top of your shoulders, so that your body carries its weight. Allowing your head to droop forward puts your neck muscles under terrific strain.
- Place a small cushion in the hollow of your back, around the level of your waist. This encourages proper posture.

Leaning forward to read or write

Since your head is the approximate weight of one of the heavier balls in a set of bowling balls – about 6 kilograms (14 pounds) – it exerts enormous strain on your neck muscles and the many small joints in that area. It is best to:

- invest in (or ask your employer to invest in) a chair that supports your whole back; if you are unable to find such a chair at normal furniture outlets, your local social services should be able to supply you with details of a specialist chair manufacturer/retailer;
- move the chair as close to the desk/table as possible to encourage proper posture;
- ensure you are sitting straight, with your bottom pressed to the back of the chair; this should prevent you from leaning forward;
- tuck in your chin as you look down, but in a relaxed manner;
- bring your work closer to eye level; you may want to use a lap desk, a drafting table, or a secure box placed on top of your regular desk or table;
- keep frequently used work materials within easy reach;
- tilt your head back every now and again to compensate for prolonged forward positioning;
- take regular breaks; if you have a lot of paperwork to get through, keep getting up and walking around;

- split the work into several short sessions; in the workplace, try to alternate 'looking down' tasks with duties where you can be more mobile.

Sitting at a keyboard

Using a keyboard can stress the joints and soft tissues in the back, neck, shoulders, arms, wrists and hands. It is best to:

- follow the above recommendations for sitting at a desk/table;
- use the computer monitor's tilting feature to find the best position; when seated, the top line of the screen should be no higher than eye level – positioning the screen too high will cause unnecessary neck strain;
- ensure that the screen is directly opposite – looking to one side for prolonged periods can severely strain the neck;
- if possible, adjust the height of your chair or work surface so your forearms are parallel with the floor and your wrists are straight; sitting at a low work surface encourages poor posture;
- invest in (or ask your employer for) a foot rest; this will reduce the pressure on your lower back;
- have the mouse and other input devices positioned so that you can use them with your arms and hands in a relaxed and natural position;
- position the keyboard directly in front of you; this makes it easier to type with your shoulders and arms relaxed;
- if you use a document holder, position it at the same level as the computer screen;
- position the mouse at the same level as the keyboard;
- keep your wrists in a straight and natural position when typing;
- keep your elbows in a relaxed position by your sides;
- purchase an ergonomic wrist support bar for your keyboard; this should help to reduce (or prevent) tendon pain – similar to that of repetitive strain injury – in your hands and wrists;
- purchase (or ask your employer to purchase) an ergonomic keyboard;
- flex your hands and wrists every ten minutes;
- if required, use a wrist splint to minimize wrist mobility;
- if using a conventional mouse, move it with your whole arm;

- use a 'moulded' mouse as this will support your hand and wrist;
- take regular breaks; you will find that frequent short breaks are far more beneficial than fewer, longer breaks;
- stand and take a few minutes to stretch your muscles between breaks;
- give yourself a time limit; when it is up, break off until later (if your pain levels begin to rise before your time is up, immediately finish what you are doing).

Reaching up to perform a task

Performing an activity while reaching upwards – for example, lifting crockery from a high shelf; replacing a light bulb; hanging curtains etc. – can put your back, shoulders and arms under enormous strain. It is best to:

- stand on a small stool (one that is very stable) so you don't have to stretch;
- use a long-handled implement for inaccessible cleaning jobs;
- take regular breaks to minimize strain;
- store items in general use – for example, groceries, pans, crockery etc. – in more accessible cupboards.

Working in the kitchen

Leaning over kitchen work surfaces for prolonged periods to wash up etc. can stress the neck and back. It is best to:

- move as close to the work surface as possible to encourage proper posture;
- stand tall, making sure to tilt your head and loosely tuck in your chin;
- place a wooden box on the work surface to bring your work closer (maybe someone keen on DIY could make you one);
- take regular breaks;
- stop as soon as you experience additional pain.

Carrying shopping, etc.

Carrying heavy shopping etc. in your hands, with your arms extended, exerts great strain on your shoulders, arms and back. It is best to:

- park as close as possible to the supermarket;
- take someone with you to share the load;
- limit the amount you carry at one time – two journeys carrying a lighter load is better than one journey carrying a heavy load;
- carry items close to your body; most Americans have the right idea where shopping is concerned – they wrap their arms around their packages because carrying objects close to the body disperses the strain;
- ensure the load is equally balanced;
- use a shopping trolley on wheels.

Lifting a bulky object off the floor

Bending your back to lift up something heavy can strain it, and your lower back is likely to be particularly vulnerable. When lifting, you should be careful to ensure your legs rather than your back take the strain. The golden rule is, therefore, LNB – Legs Not Back. Don't forget to assess, first of all, whether you are really up to lifting. If you choose to go ahead, it is best to:

- plant your feet about 30 cm (12 in) or so apart, as a wide base helps to maintain correct alignment;
- keep your back straight, bend your knees until you are resting on your haunches, and place your arms around the object;
- push upwards with your legs in order to raise the object from the ground;
- break the load, if possible, into smaller 'portions'; where laundry is concerned, it is safer to lift a few items at a time – carrying them close to your body (perhaps over your arm if the items are dry) to the washing machine/tumble drier/ clothes airer;
- get someone to help if the object is larger than a laundry basket.

Carrying a bulky object

Carrying can severely stress the muscles and joints in the hands, wrists, arms, shoulders, neck and back. It is best to:

- keep the object close to your body as you walk, and ensure your grip is firm;

- maintain an upright posture, again ensuring that your legs – not your back – take the strain (LNB);
- rest the object on an available surface – that is, a table or work surface – to give your muscles a break during carrying.

Setting down a bulky object

Placing a bulky object on the floor stresses the lower back in particular. It is best to:

- plant your feet about 30 cm (12 in) apart;
- keep your back straight, bend your knees, and let your legs take the strain as you lower the object to the floor (LNB);
- put the laundry basket on a nearby patio table/garden bench or a broad-topped wall if you are transporting laundry, for example, from the kitchen to the outside washing line; putting the laundry basket down will save you the strain of lowering it to the ground.

Picking up something light off the floor

Most people tend to arch right over to pick up a piece of fluff, for example, from the carpet. This can put enormous strain on the back – in particular, the lower back. It is best to:

- keep your back straight, and bend your knees until you are able to reach the object;
- use your thigh muscles to propel you upright again (LNB);
- use a long-handled 'grabber' if your hips and legs are too painful to do the above.

Bending forward to perform a task

Bending to push laundry into the washing machine or put a dish into a free-standing oven can stress your back and shoulders. It is best to:

- lower yourself into a kneeling position, keeping your back straight;
- push in only a small amount of washing at a time; several repetitions are better than thrusting in one great bundle at once (reverse the procedure to remove the washing).

Lying in bed all night

Lying down for long periods can make you feel stiff and sore. It is best to:

- never sleep on your stomach;
- when lying on your back, place a pillow beneath your knees to minimize the strain on your lower back;
- use no more than one small pillow to support your head and neck – moulded cervical pillows keep the head correctly aligned during sleep;
- turn on to your side to relieve the pressure on your back, and place a pillow between your knees to take the strain off your hips;
- use a reasonably firm mattress; mattresses that sag will contribute to your problems.

Driving the car

Driving can stress virtually every muscle in the body. It is therefore important always to assess whether you are up to driving before you set out. If you believe you are, it is best to:

- adjust the seat so it is near the steering column;
- make sure the back of the seat is adjusted correctly; it should be neither too upright, nor too far reclined;
- not slouch or allow your head to droop forwards;
- wear an inflatable neck support;
- use a lumbar support (a cushion in the small of your back will do);
- ensure your car has a headrest. In the unlucky event of a collision, the headrest can minimize the severity of whiplash injury;
- use armrests when driving – these reduce stress on the arms, shoulders and upper back; armrests can also help to support the upper back when you are travelling as a passenger;
- use your wing mirrors to facilitate reversing;
- opt for power steering, if possible, when changing your car; if your purse doesn't stretch to this, make sure you perform

plenty of slow manoeuvres when you take a car for a test drive – then pick a car with light steering (some small cars can be surprisingly heavy to handle at slow speeds);

- choose, when buying a new car, one with an automatic gearbox; this will eliminate the need to constantly depress the clutch and shift the gear stick;
- have power-controlled windows, wing mirrors, sun-roof etc. as these are easier to manage than their manually controlled counterparts;
- make regular breaks in a long journey to walk around and stretch your muscles;
- share the driving with someone else;
- apply for a Blue Badge to enable you to park closer to your destination, in a specially designated disabled parking space; the badge can be used in any privately owned vehicle in which you are travelling – for example, if you are being driven to the shops by a neighbour;
- use the train and claim Attendance Allowance (if you are unable to drive), and apply for a Disabled Person's Railcard (valid throughout the UK) which discounts the usual cost by about a third;
- have a specially adapted car if necessary; you will need to contact an accredited driving assessment centre with regard to this. Once your car has been adapted (or you have purchased one that has already been adapted), you must inform the Driver Vehicle Licensing Agency (DVLA). If your arthritis affects your ability to drive in any way, you must also inform your insurance company.

Rising from a chair

Thrusting your upper body forward in order to get out of your seat can stress the muscles of your entire back. It is best to:

- move your bottom to the edge of the seat;
- place one foot as far backwards as possible;
- use the armrests to help propel you upwards, making sure you don't lean forward as you stand up.

Getting out of bed

Twisting your body to get out of bed (or off the sofa) can put your back and hips under a lot of strain. It is best to:

- roll on to your side (if you are not already on it) and push the duvet back;
- move your knees forward so they hang slightly over the bed edge;
- swing your feet outwards and over the edge of the bed;
- place the palm of your overhead arm on the bed at the level of your waist and as you push your body upwards, and swing your legs down until they touch the floor. This should smoothly propel you into a sitting position.

Useful addresses

UK and continental Europe

Arthritis Care
18 Stephenson Way
London NW1 2HD
Tel.: 020 7380 6500
Helpline (freephone): 0808 800 4050 (10 a.m. to 4 p.m., Monday to Friday)
Website: www.arthritiscare.org.uk

Arthritis Research UK
Copeman House
St Mary's Gate
Chesterfield
Derbyshire S41 7TD
Tel.: 01246 558033
Website: www.arthritisresearchuk.org

As well as funding research, Arthritis Research UK produces a range of free information booklets and leaflets.

Carers UK
20 Great Dover Street
London SE1 4LX
Tel.: 020 7378 4999
Fax: 020 7378 9781
Website: www.carersuk.org

Carers UK is the voice of carers. The association gives support to those who provide unpaid care by looking after an ill, frail or disabled family member, friend or partner.

CherryActive
99 Manor Lane
Sunbury
Middlesex TW16 6JE
Tel.: 08451 705705
Website: www.cherryactive.co.uk

Cherry Active juice and capsules are available for purchase from the website.

Children's Chronic Arthritis Association (CCAA)
Ground Floor
Amber Gate City Wall Road
Worcester WR1 2AH

Tel.: 01905 745595
Website: www.ccaa.org.uk

Offers advice and support for the families of children with juvenile arthritis.

Fibromyalgia Association UK
PO Box 206
Stourbridge DY9 8YL
Tel. (helpline): 0845 345 2322 (10 a.m. to 4 p.m., Monday to Friday)
Helpline for fibromyalgia-related benefit advice (run by Mrs Janet Horton, a trustee of the Association): 0870 751 7389 (10 a.m. to midday, Mondays and Fridays)
Fax: 01384 895005
Website: www.fibromyalgia-associationuk.org

The Fibromyalgia Association UK is a registered charity administered by unpaid volunteers. It was established to provide information and support to people with fibromyalgia and their families. In addition, the Association provides medical information for professionals and operates a national helpline.

Fibromyalgia Support Northern Ireland (FMSNI)
The Vine Centre
193 Crumlin Road
Belfast BT14 7DX
Northern Ireland
Helpline: 0844 826 9024 (10.30 a.m. to 4 p.m., Monday to Friday)
Text: 07549 838800 (for urgent enquiries when out and about)
Website: www.fmsni.org.uk

This organization is dedicated to raising awareness of fibromyalgia and supporting people with the condition.

Green Ways International
Tel. (mobile): 00 34 686 739 300 (ask for Madhu)
Email: mdhankani25@yahoo.com

For good quality barley grass juice products at reasonable prices.

National Rheumatoid Arthritis Society (NRAS)
Unit B4, Westacott Business Centre
Westacott Way
Littlewick Green
Maidenhead
Berkshire SL6 3RT
Tel. (freephone helpline): 0800 298 7650
Website: www.nras.org.uk

Provides information and support for people with rheumatoid arthritis and their families.

Nutri Centre
Unit 3, Kendal Court
Kendal Avenue
London W3 0RU
Tel.: 0845 602 6744 (for mail order and general enquiries; mail order available 9 a.m. to 6 p.m., Monday to Friday; 10 a.m. to 4 p.m., Saturdays)
Website: www.nutricentre.com

For good quality vitamins, minerals and supplements.

UK Fibromyalgia (associated with the **Fibromyalgia Association UK**)
7 Ashbourne Road
Bournemouth
Dorset BH5 2JS
Tel. and Fax: 01202 259155
Website: www.ukfibromyalgia.com

Offers fibromyalgia-related information and advice, experts' comments and more. The site also publishes the monthly *FaMily* magazine.

Vitamins Direct
Goldshield Ltd
NLS Tower
12–16 Addiscombe Road
Croydon
Surrey CRO OXT
Tel. (freephone): 0800 634 9985 (8 a.m. to 8 p.m. daily)
Website: http://vitaminsdirect.co.uk

Vitamins Direct is a leading supplier of good-quality vitamins, minerals and supplements.

Weight Watchers (UK) Ltd
Millennium House
Ludlow Road
Maidenhead
Berkshire SL6 2SL
Tel.: 0845 345 1500
Website: www.weightwatchers.co.uk

For details of WeightWatchers meetings in the UK, go to the website or write to the above address.

USA

American Juvenile Arthritis Organization (AJAO) see Arthritis Foundation

Arthritis Foundation
PO Box 7669
Atlanta, GA 30357-0669
USA
Tel.: +1 800 283 7800
Website: www.arthritis.org

Gives support and information to people with arthritis and their families and carers. The **American Juvenile Arthritis Organization (AJAO)**, a Council of the Arthritis Foundation, is dedicated to providing information and advice to the parents of children with juvenile arthritis.

National Fibromyalgia Association
2121 S. Towne Centre Place
Suite 300
Anaheim, CA 92806
USA
Tel.: +1 714 921 0150
Website: www.fmaware.org

This members-only website gives information on support groups and fibromyalgia-related community events from Canada to California. The Association also publishes the monthly *Fibromyalgia AWARE* magazine.

Notes

1 Martin, K. R. *et al.*, 'The role of pain intensity and pain limitation as mediators in the relationship between arthritis status and seven psychosocial health outcomes', abstract presented at the American College of Rheumatology Annual Scientific Meeting, San Francisco, October 2008.
2 Clegg, D. O. *et al.*, 'Glucosamine, chondroitin sulphate and the two in combination for painful knee osteoarthritis', *New England Journal of Medicine*, 354: 795–808, 2006.

Further reading

Craggs-Hinton, Christine, *Coping with Gout*, Sheldon Press, 2004 (new edn 2011).

Craggs-Hinton, Christine, *Living with Fibromyalgia*, Sheldon Press, 2010.

Doyle, Penny, and Deane, Audrey, *The Top 100 Omega-3 Recipes: Reduce Your Risk of Heart Disease, Keep Your Brain Active and Agile*, Duncan Baird Publishers, 2009.

Green, Wendy, *50 Things You Can Do To Manage Arthritis*, Summersdale, 2010.

Hills, Margaret, *Treating Arthritis Exercise Book*, Sheldon Press, 2010.

Holford, Patrick, *Say No to Arthritis: The Proven Drug Free Guide to Preventing and Relieving Arthritis*, Piatkus Books, 1999.

Jenkins, Jasmine, *How to Live a Full Life with Rheumatoid Arthritis: How to Manage Your Rheumatoid Arthritis by Becoming an Expert Patient*, How To Books, 2008.

Patten, Marguerite, and Ewin, Jeannette, *Eat to Beat Arthritis: Over 60 Recipes and a Self-treatment Plan to Transform Your Life*, Thorsons, 2004.

Wall, Patrick, and Melzack, Ronald, *The Challenge of Pain* (Penguin Science), Penguin, 2008.

Weil, Andrew, *Eating Well for Optimum Health: The Essential Guide to Food, Diet and Nutrition*, Sphere, 2008.

Index